Yoga in Practice

Also by Katy Appleton

Introducing Yoga

Yoga in Practice

A Complete System to Tone the Body,
Bring Emotional Balance
and Promote Good Health

Katy Appleton

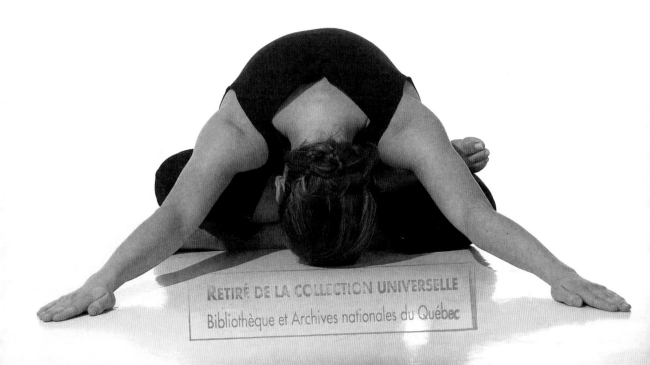

MACMILLAN

First published 2004 by Macmillan
an imprint of Pan Macmillan Publishers Ltd
Pan Macmillan, 20 New Wharf Road, London N1 9RR
Basingstoke and Oxford
Associated companies throughout the world
www.panmacmillan.com

ISBN 1 4050 0550 5

1 3 5 7 9 8 6 4 2

A CIP catalogue record for this book is available from
the British Library.

Photography by Jim Marks
Illustrations © Becky Hall
Design by Louise Millar
Printed and bound by Butler and Tanner

Contents

Foreword by Narayani and Barbara Gordon   7

INTRODUCTION
The Experience of Yoga   8
How to Use this Book   9

A BRIEF HISTORY OF YOGA
The Four Pathways of Yoga   12

YOGA OF THE MIND, BODY AND SPIRIT
Introduction to Hatha Yoga   17
Breathing   20
Relaxation   30
Sun Salutation   35
Standing Postures   43
Floor Postures   81
Backward Bending Postures   105
Inverted Postures   128
Meditation   163
Chakras and the Energetic Body   171
Mudras   174
The Yoga of Sound   176

HOW TO BUILD YOUR OWN PRACTICE
General Guidelines   180
Building a Class   182
The Postures and Their Benefits Chart   188

Final Thoughts   190

About Katy Appleton   192

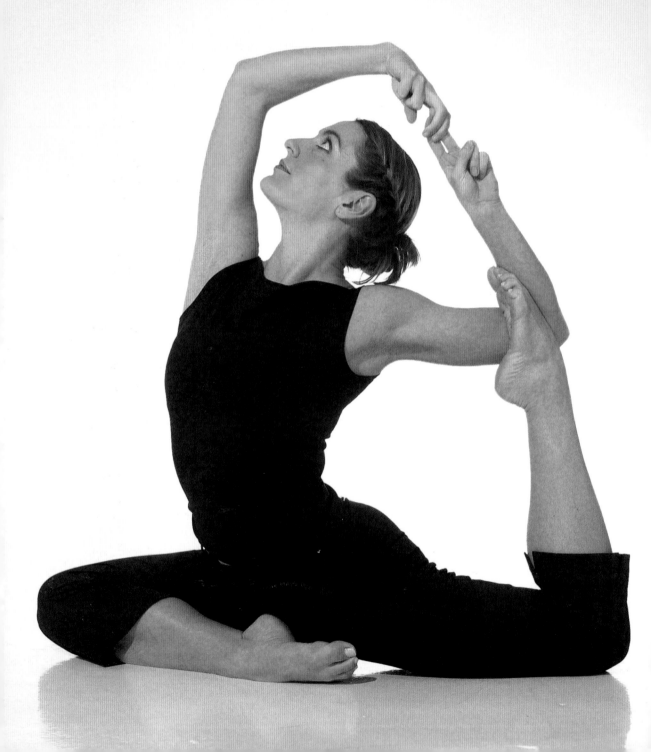

For my mum
Who is always in my heart

Foreword

I invited my first yoga teachers, Narayani and Barbara Gordon, to write the opening words of my book.

The science of yoga has been written about for a long long time, originally in brief phrases designed for easy recall and commentary by the teacher.

The yogi asks, 'Who am I?' and spends his life seeking to understand, to realize his true nature.

'We can't help being thirsty, moving towards the voice of water' – Rumi.

The word for spiritual practice, sadhana, means striving. To the yogi, life is sadhana, life is striving after this essential truth behind 'Who am I?' Often we ask, 'Who is asking, who am I?' and this forms the basis of one of the niyamas, the observances of Raja Yoga: swadhaya, or self-study, for yoga is truly introspectional psychology.

Reading, as you are now, is a valid form of swadhaya. Observe your own responses to the thoughts presented, and use those as stepping stones to go within. Find the thoughts that resonate with you and go back to them again and again, savouring these thoughts in your meditation and, indeed, during your asanas.

Some days when you're unsure how to begin, simply open your book at random and meditate on what comes up. We truly live in wonderful times, with so much inspiration available to us. Katy's writing is cheerful, encouraging and accessible, based on her personal experience as a modern yogi.

So, dear reader, in your sadhana, whatever else you discover yourself to be – be a yogi.

Narayani

Yoga has become known in the West as a form of exercise, or as something cultish. It is neither. It is an entire science and way of life incorporating exercise, lifestyle, a way of thinking and being leading ultimately to what the yogis call samahdi, self-knowledge or realization. To be at peace with yourself, without desire, totally in the present, not regretting the past or living in the future.

Everyone on this planet wants happiness and contentment. In the west people are continuously looking outside of themselves to achieve this: through another person, material gain, a bigger house, more money, and so on. This is ultimately useless as the only true happiness in this life lies within. Nothing of a material nature can ever satisfy what we truly are searching for, and that is peace of mind.

The path to true happiness lies within and however much you try to disprove this you will see ultimately it is a pointless task to look outside yourself for what is staring us in the face and within our grasp.

I wish you all a successful journey on this exciting path of yoga and am sure Katy's book will offer inspiration to one and all who read it.

Barbara Gordon

Introduction

The Experience of Yoga

Yoga brings me a deep sense of peace, the feeling that I am returning home, and a happiness I want to share with you. I hope that through this book you will find your own joy. Yoga is an experiment with the self. It gives us many different tools and techniques to work with to uncover our true potential as humans – that is, as joyful spiritual beings. If you love to move then you may be drawn to the physical side of yoga first, or if you are intrigued by how your mind works the meditational and introspective side of yoga may appeal. There are many different pathways to follow in yoga – choose your gateway in, knowing that eventually it will lead you, and all that practise, to the same place: bliss.

I came to yoga before I was born – my mother did yoga classes while she was pregnant. Then I went along with her to a few yoga classes as a small child. From an early age my path was obvious: I just wanted to move. I felt it from deep within, the need to dance, to express myself through movement. After many years of disciplined and dedicated practice I became a professional ballet dancer. I adored it. To be on stage allowed me to experience being totally present in the moment. Looking back, I can see I was practising yoga even then. I was so absorbed by the steps I was dancing and the movement of my body flowing with the music that there was no space for my mind to wander off. This is what yoga means: union, to connect one's mind, body and spirit in the present moment.

It was obvious to me from early on as a dancer that I needed to balance the physical work somehow. Instinctively, I started to sit quietly for periods of time, observing my breath. This made me feel calm and created the balance in life I felt I needed.

Looking back it's interesting to see that I was practising some of the techniques of yoga without realizing it. I'm sure this is the case with many people. Anyway, I attended a yoga class with a friend one day and was amazed at how I felt at the end of the practice. I couldn't believe how an hour and a half of postures could make me feel so euphoric. I was hooked. To begin with, my practice was all physical. It felt very natural, as a dancer, to experiment with my body, but as my practice developed I soon realized that yoga was so much more than a set of physical postures and this really intrigued me. I began to feel a calmness within that made me view my outside world with different eyes. I realized that yoga kept me balanced and that I needed yoga in my life. At that point I decided to train to teach yoga so that I could absorb myself daily in its treasures and convey them to others. My hope is that by writing this book you will begin to understand the vast potential that resides within each and every one of us – potential for change, for growth, for knowledge, and for happiness and contentment. Namaste.

How to Use this Book

This book will take you through the physical and spiritual benefits yoga can bring. Yoga can stretch, tone and strengthen your body, alleviate physical ailments, reduce stress and bring greater mental clarity. Yoga has all the tools and techniques needed to do any work on the mind, body and breath. Knowing the best way to use these tools is something that can only be achieved through practice, experience, trial and error. As a yoga teacher I also understand that, for the average person, physical flexibility can be a real problem. This should never be a deterrent to the practice of yoga. In fact, the more you practise the postures the more the body becomes supple and strong. Besides, even the most advanced yogis have flexibility problems; theirs might just be a bit more complex!

For those who are completely new to yoga, and, more importantly, for those who do not have any system of personal exercise, I recommend reading my first book, *Introducing Yoga*, in order to begin to understand how yoga views the physical and mental body. That book concentrates on warm-up exercises, which might be helpful if you have little or no experience of moving your body in this way. The practice of yoga postures really is for everyone, but some basic flexibility is necessary. If you have any doubts about your fitness or capabilities, whether because of a prior injury or age or anything at all, please consult your doctor or a certified yoga teacher. If yoga is approached with complete awareness it will be hugely beneficial for anyone, whatever age or physical condition, but without having the benefit of guiding you in person it is very difficult for me to tell you what you should or shouldn't do. I will point out potential dangers and try to highlight common mistakes, but please always listen to your own body and approach yoga without any sense of competition. Yoga is all about you, not anyone else. The greatest and most satisfying achievements are those you did not think possible, and as long as you relax and allow yourself to enjoy testing your own physical and mental limitations, the benefits you gain from yoga will be enormous.

I am only a guide on your own personal journey. In opening this book you have joined millions of others who have turned to yoga to bring greater peace and happiness to their lives. As a teacher of this ancient practice, I am simply a pathway through which the teachings of many before me can be brought to you. By experimenting with the techniques you will figure out the best way yoga can help you. I will give you ideas and hints based on my own practise and experience as a teacher, but I leave it to you to explore your own body and mind freely.

Here's a brief outline of what you'll find in the rest of the book:

A Brief History of Yoga is an introduction to four paths that make up yoga and shows you how the physical postures fit into the vast science of yoga.

The next chapter is Yoga of the Mind, Body and Spirit. The most commonly seen and taught form of yoga is Hatha Yoga, physical yoga. In this section I will take you through breathing and relaxation techniques and a wide range of physical postures. The physical postures are graded and I recommend that you start with the simpler ones (level 1) and only move on to the more challenging ones once you are fully comfortable with the basics. The majority of injuries occur when students practising yoga try to achieve postures beyond their capabilities at that time. Never let your ego dictate how much you attempt. Listen to your body – I promise you it will be your guide. If it tells you to stop something that feels uncomfortable, then please don't ignore the message. Yoga is also a discipline of the mind as much as the body, so I have also included a chapter on meditation. Yoga also views the body in an energetic way, so I thought it would be interesting to write a simple explanation of the chakras, what mudras are and how chanting can uplift and energize our mind, body and spirit.

The final chapter, How to Build Your Own Practice, covers the basic principles you can follow in order to sequence your postures and build a practice that fulfils the goals you have set. A proper physical yoga practice should work each set of muscles in every direction, stretching and contracting in almost equal measure. Once you understand the principles of sequencing, balance, counterbalance and moving through the body, you should be able to design your own practice with relative ease. This chapter is likely to answer questions you might have and so I recommend you read the book through to the end before you experiment with any of the postures.

Finally, I recommend that you read everything in this book at least once. A lot of the ideas become clearer the more understanding you have of yoga as a whole. Take your time and try to absorb as much information as possible before starting to put it all into practice. After all, you are in no hurry. Be patient, and the rewards will be revealed to you exactly when they are supposed to be.

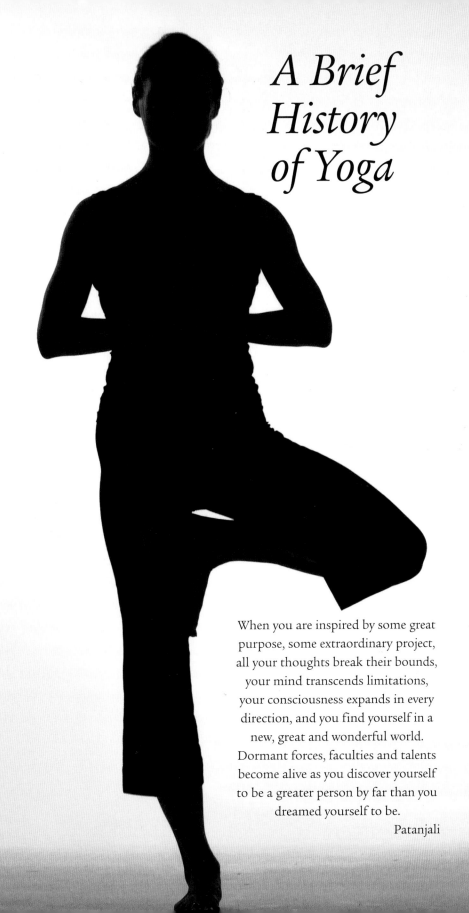

A Brief History of Yoga

When you are inspired by some great purpose, some extraordinary project, all your thoughts break their bounds, your mind transcends limitations, your consciousness expands in every direction, and you find yourself in a new, great and wonderful world. Dormant forces, faculties and talents become alive as you discover yourself to be a greater person by far than you dreamed yourself to be.

Patanjali

The Four Pathways of Yoga

Yoga as we know it today was developed thousands of years ago in the Indus Valley of ancient northern India. Archaeological digs made in this area have uncovered statues depicting deities that resemble Lord Shiva, the mythical and legendary teacher of yoga, in various postures (*asanas*) and practising meditation. Some of these might be up to ten thousand years old. During this period yoga techniques were never written down. Instead they were passed down from teacher (*guru*) to student (*sadhaka*) through personal instruction. In this way the guru could control the flow of information to the student in order to ensure clear understanding. Yoga was generally used as a tool for intense meditation so that individuals could realize their spiritual potential, and the asanas that developed through the centuries grew as a response to the increased awareness that a healthy body was essential for long periods of meditation. It is for this reason that nearly all yoga postures influence the spine in some way or another. For a person sitting cross-legged in meditation for long periods, a strong and supple spine is of great importance.

The system of yoga can be thought of as a great tree, with the various branches representing the different pathways of yoga, which all lead to the same goal: the supreme state of liberation. The yoga that we most often see practised in the west, involving movement of the body coordinated with precise breathing, is part of Raja Yoga, one of the four main branches that make up the tree of yoga.

The Tree of Yoga

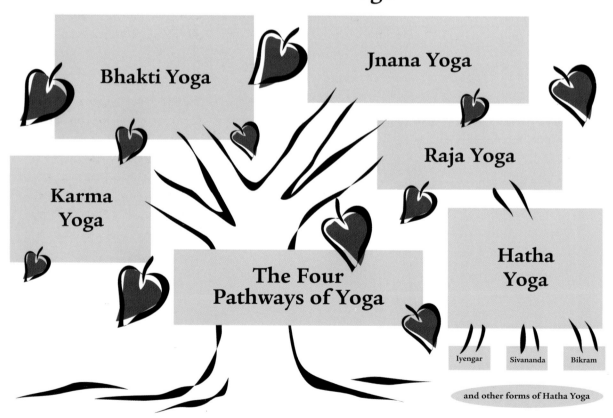

Bhakti Yoga

Jnana Yoga

Raja Yoga

Karma Yoga

The Four Pathways of Yoga

Hatha Yoga

Iyengar   Sivananda   Bikram

and other forms of Hatha Yoga

Karma Yoga

The word *karma* may be translated as 'action'. Every thought, word and deed bears fruit, whether in this life or in subsequent lives. You can never be certain exactly how karma will manifest, all you can be sure of is that your actions will have consequences. The quality of the present action (thought, word or deed) determines the quality of the future circumstance. The path of Karma Yoga is the path of selfless service, of performing actions without any thought of gain or reward. Through the complete indifference to all desires or gain, you are able to become closer to your divine and perfect state. Observe and be aware of the intentions behind every action you perform, and you may see that the ideal of Karma Yoga is a far greater challenge to achieve than may first appear.

Bhakti Yoga

Bhakti can be translated as 'devotion'. In traditional yoga, the object of your devotion would almost certainly be God, or at least a form of God. In traditional Indian Hinduism there are many forms of God, each representing a different facet of the divine spirit. For instance, in India you will find followers of Shiva, Vishnu, Brahma, Ganesha and many more. Each of these deities is unique but each represents part of the same ultimate God. However, provided that your devotion is inspired by pure love, then the object of your adoration could be just about anything. For instance, you could easily imagine devoting your life to the pure nature of every human spirit on the planet. Whenever we use prayer, worship, ritual or chanting to unconditionally surrender ourselves to a higher spirit or ideal, devoting our thoughts and deeds to that higher force, then we bring Bhakti Yoga into our lives.

Jnana Yoga

Jnana Yoga is the path of knowledge and wisdom, and those who have practised it can be compared with some of the great philosophical thinkers of the western world. This path requires great strength of will and intellect, and encourages the yogi to use his or her own mind to enquire into the nature of life and everything. According to yoga philosophy, we are one with God, inseparable from the divine. However, in our ignorance (*avidya*) we are unaware of our own divine nature and so create a world of conflict. Jnana Yoga seeks to break down the barriers of ignorance in our mind through inquiry, introspection and deep contemplation and meditation. By removing false ideas about who we are, we shed conditioning and become a true expression of divinity.

Raja Yoga

This is the science of physical and mental control, the 'royal' yoga, a complete method for turning mental and physical energy into a far greater force: spiritual. A sage called Patanjali formally systematized the path of Raja Yoga by detailing it precisely in his *Yoga Sutras*. Patanjali's Raja Yoga system is about creating peace of mind, about being connected to, and surrendering to, the joyful, harmonious flow of life. If taken up as a spiritual practice it results in freedom, liberation and self-acceptance. When you are peaceful and calm within, you will experience the outside world with clarity. You can go through life content, the mind unoccupied by trivial matters, seeing beyond the small world of personal desires. The path he proposed to achieve these states is often known as Astanga Yoga, the 'eight-limb path'. (There is some confusion surrounding the word *astanga*, mainly because of the westernized form of Hatha Yoga (physical yoga) that is also known as Astanga – or Ashtanga – Yoga. Although this Hatha Yoga form takes its name from the classical eight-limb path of Patanjali, in practice it has very little to do with Patanjali's *Yoga Sutras*.)

The Eight-limb Path

The eight limbs of Patanjali's system are yama, niyama, asana, pranayama, pratyahara, dharana, dhyana and samadhi.

Yama and Niyama

The yamas and niyamas are ethical and spiritual practices. The five yamas are ethical foundations for living one's life. *Ahimsa* (non-violence) is having consideration for all beings and living in a way that causes as little harm as possible. *Satya* (truth) is about approaching the world with pure intentions. *Asteya* (non-stealing) is to take only what is freely given, to take only what we need in life, to live simply. *Bramacharya* (sexual conduct) is about redirecting rather than wasting our sexual energy and transforming it towards spiritual purposes. *Aparigraha* (non-greed) is being able to step back, to watch and observe what we grasp for.

The five niyamas are more internally focused. *Saucha* (purity) is to engage in things that are purifying. *Santosha* is practising contentment in life. *Tapas* (discipline) is a conscious commitment to an aim and staying with it through all distracting desires and obstacles. *Swadhaya* (self-study) is getting to know the self – we have much potential in life but we can't use it without the ability to see inside ourselves. *Ishvara pranidhana* (devotion) is to take shelter in the supreme state.

The practice of the yamas and niyamas is the foundation for attaining Patanjali's state of peaceful mind. It is not necessary to practise them all at once; in fact, it might be overwhelming to do so. The key is to look at the various ways each of them can be interpreted and applied to your life. Eventually, through experience you will see how the yamas and niyamas overlap and carry each other – and support you in unshakeable peace of mind. Take time to practise them and you will find increasing independence and happiness, free from public opinion and peer pressure. In short, you will begin to discover who you really are.

Asana and Pranayama

In the *Yoga Sutras* the word *asana* refers to a 'steady and comfortable' pose for meditation. *Pranayama* is described as the control (or restraint) of the breath, or *kumbhaka*. Asana and pranayama are both part of the practice of Hatha Yoga, or physical yoga, the form of Yoga most commonly seen and taught in the west. Under the generic umbrella of Hatha Yoga there are many different methods to choose from, such as Iyengar, Sivananda, Bikram and Astanga, to name but a few. Find a method or methods that suit you but know that, in the larger picture of yoga, these techniques are preparation for the body and mind to be able to sit still and comfortably for long periods of time. If the body is stiff and unyielding, if the breathing is shallow and stunted, how can anyone go deeper within?

Pratyahara, Dharana, Dhyana and Samadhi

Once you are able to sit still and comfortably, by closing your eyes you can withdraw into your internal world (*pratyahara*) and concentrate (*dharana*). There are many techniques to achieve a state of complete concentration and I will give you a few examples to experiment with in the section on meditation.

Once you have succeeded in fully emptying your mind of all distractions and focused on the object of concentration, you have then entered into a state of *dhyana*, proper meditation. This is a peaceful and calm state of being where time seems to stand still and only you and the object of your concentration exist, free of any effort. In that moment there will be no need to be anywhere else. No desires invade your mind, no distractions occur and you will arrive in the state of complete absorption in the current moment: *samadhi*.

There is no need to be religious to enjoy the benefits of yoga. Except for practice of Bhakti Yoga, there is no necessity for any kind of faith or belief in God or any higher power. Yoga is more scientific, requiring experimentation with its theories and practices in the individual's search for the truth, although you may find that continued and deep practice of yoga reveals a spiritual side that was previously hidden.

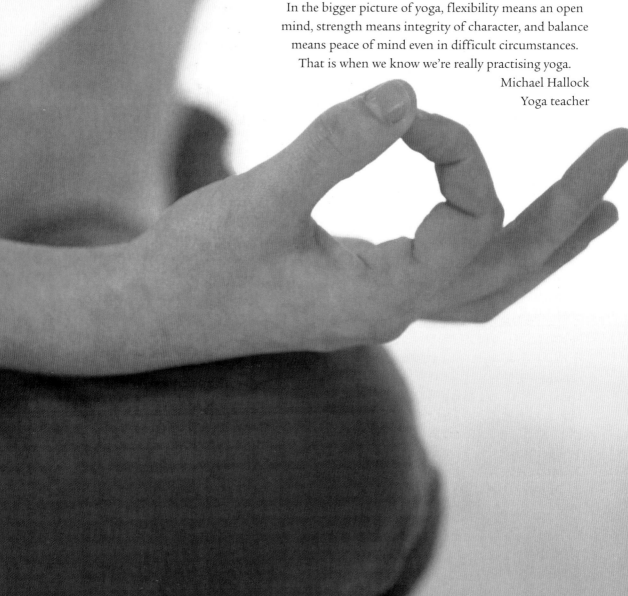

Yoga of the Mind, Body and Spirit

True progress in yoga means more than physical
accomplishments of flexibility, strength and balance.
In the bigger picture of yoga, flexibility means an open
mind, strength means integrity of character, and balance
means peace of mind even in difficult circumstances.
That is when we know we're really practising yoga.

Michael Hallock
Yoga teacher

Introduction to Hatha Yoga

This is the core of the book. The section covers a large number of the most common postures in yoga, as well as breathing and relaxation techniques. Reading and understanding the breathing and relaxation techniques first will help you with all the physical postures later.

The Sanskrit word for postures, *asana*, translates as a 'steady, comfortable pose'. Although I will use the word 'posture' (or 'pose') in this text, and not 'asana', the definition should be remembered throughout. Try to practise all the postures and breathing techniques in a relaxed state with as little tension as possible. Obviously in some of the more advanced postures there will be some tension in the body. However, as much as you can, try to visualize the mind and body in states such as 'ease', 'relaxation', 'softness' and 'enjoyment' when in any posture. Try to challenge yourself from one session to another, too, remembering where your limitations were and trying to move further into the postures and breathing techniques each time you try them. Although such progressions may be very subtle, added up over time they will produce noticeable and lasting improvements in your strength, flexibility and breath. You may not be able to see external progress all the time but that does not mean nothing is happening. Often the greatest progress is that which we cannot see: internal changes to the body over time that appear externally when you least expect it.

How to Read the Postures

Take your time to read and understand the text for each posture and breathing technique. Read and re-read the descriptions – even after practising, continue to read the descriptions to help you to go deeper and deeper into the movements and breath. This is how the descriptions appear.

The Name
The English name given for each posture and breathing technique is the most common name used for that pose. Different schools of yoga may use other names, so don't be concerned if you hear someone describing a posture using a different name to the one you know. This is also the case with the Sanskrit names of the postures and breathing techniques (given in brackets). In this section you will also find a rating for each posture (though not for the breathing techniques). The ratings are:
1 Beginners
2 Intermediate
3 Advanced
Please be aware that for some of the more advanced postures (2–3 or 3), beginner's variations may be given. Remember that the beginner's variation of an advanced pose will still be regarded as advanced in itself, and should only be attempted when you are ready for that level.

The Technique

Read the description at least once before trying the posture or breathing technique, and then come back to the text as often as you need, because there are a lot of points to take on all at once. (This is especially the case for some of the visualizations. Everybody sees things in different ways, so don't worry if you have trouble seeing some of the visualizations I have suggested.) I am only a guide. If you find you have a better way to do or think about a posture, go for it. You are the best judge of your own body. Variations on a posture, either for beginners or more advanced students, are highlighted in shaded boxes.

Benefits

These are the most common benefits, based on my own knowledge gained through teaching and reading. There may be other benefits. If you discover some I have not mentioned, please feel free to email me about them (see address on page 192). I am always interested in learning more about how yoga affects different people.

Common Mistakes

These are the most common mistakes I have seen as a teacher. These should give you a good idea of what to avoid. Read and re-read them, and try to apply the knowledge in each posture.

Contraindications

Here I list specific contraindications. If you have an injury that affects certain movements, listen to what your body is telling you and use your common sense as to what you can and cannot do.

Sequence

The suggestions given here are very general. I discuss the principles of sequencing much more in the chapter How To Build Your Own Practice. Breathing techniques should always be done together, so there is no sequence advice in the Breathing section.

Awareness

Physical awareness: Suggested parts of the body to think about during each posture and breathing technique. You may find other areas to think about based on your own abilities.

Energetic awareness: For those who want to incorporate chakra visualizations into their practice. This is one of the last layers to add to your practice, and only after you are fully relaxed and comfortable in the posture. If you want to try it, choose a posture or breathing technique you can do in comfort, then think about some of the elements of the chakra associated with it, such as its colour or location.

Ten Top Practice Tips

1. Before anything else, learn to breathe correctly. In all my beginner's courses the first areas I cover are the abdominal and yogic breathing techniques. The realization of proper breathing is often one of the most surprising and wonderful aspects of yoga practice.

2. Use a proper yoga mat. There is a real risk of slipping on any other surface. Wear comfortable clothes that your body can move freely in. Yoga is normally practised in bare feet.

3. Leave a minimum of two hours after eating before practising.

4. Create a relaxing atmosphere. Maybe light a candle, some incense or an aromatherapy oil burner.

5. Turn off your telephones and TV. Gentle music in the background can be inspiring, although for some it is a distraction. Find what works for you each time you practise. Don't let anyone disturb you; this time is for you and you alone.

6. Try to create some space in your home where you can practise every day. If you can keep your mat on the floor all the time do so, as this will remind you to step on it to practise.

7. To start with, set yourself a goal to practise yoga for 10–15 minutes daily; everybody has time for that. Then gradually build up to a longer practice that fits in with your life. Eventually your practice will become part of your everyday routine and, like brushing your teeth, you'll know when you have missed it.

8. If you have any longstanding injuries or illnesses, please consult your doctor before you begin to practise yoga. This book is not written with pregnancy in mind, although yoga during pregnancy is wonderful. If you wish to practise yoga during pregnancy I would suggest that you find a qualified teacher.

9. The mind loves to wander to the past or future – try to stay in the present moment. It helps to keep the mind on the breath, observing what it is doing and how it feels. By doing this, the mind stays in the now.

10. Be aware of how you are feeling each time you start your practice. It will always be different; sometimes the energy is high, sometimes it is low. Listen to what your body is telling you and adjust your practice to suit. There is no competition in yoga, with yourself or with others. All you need is a certain willingness to try, patience in your learning, awareness and concentration in order to progress, and happiness in all you do!

Breathing

The morning wind spreads its fresh smell,
We must get up and take that in,
That wind that lets us live,
Breathe before it's gone.

Rumi

Without the breath there would be no human life to speak of. Despite its obvious importance in maintaining life, the breath is something many of us do unconsciously, as if there was no need to nurture and care for it. So our breathing habits become poor, and the majority of us use only a small part of our full lung capacity in our normal inhalation and exhalation.

In yoga the breath is equal to the energy of life. Inhalations are not just a matter of allowing oxygen into our system. A proper inhalation also brings energy, inspiration, light and nourishment from the universe into our body and soul. Neither are the exhalations just a tool to expel waste from our system. Exhalations give something back to the universe, get rid of negativity and stress, and allow you to clean your body internally. Control of breathing concentrates the vital nerve energy, leading to increased control of the body and mind. Even modern medicine acknowledges the importance of proper breathing.

The link between the body and the breath is obvious enough. The muscles need oxygen constantly. When we exercise, the muscles require even more oxygen than usual, more than normal breathing provides, and so we quicken the breath. In yoga, however, we learn that this quickening of the breath does not necessarily provide the extra oxygen – most of us simply inhale and exhale more quickly rather than take in more oxygen. Proper breathing is about feeling the movement of the inhalation build up deep in the diaphragm, then slowly and just as deeply exhaling. This pushes the new energy throughout your body as well as expelling waste from your lungs. By controlling the breath you will find that you receive all the extra oxygen your muscles require without having to quicken the breath or stop the activity you are doing.

We also know of the link between the mind and the breath, although we may not always be aware of it. When we concentrate deeply on the breath it tends to slow down and lengthen; it may stop entirely for a time. Likewise, when we are agitated or bothered, the breath speeds up, becomes shallow and disjointed. The breath acts as a bridge from mind to body – and vice versa. By slowing the breath and consciously controlling the inhalation and exhalation, we are able to clear the mind and listen to the rhythm of the body, the pulse of the universe.

The techniques shown here are by no means advanced, and may be practised by anyone. The benefits to be gained from taking time to be aware of how you breathe are enormous. Give yourself 10 minutes or so to try these techniques and continue to practise them as often as possible. Over time you will discover that sinus problems are alleviated, breathing becomes deeper and more natural, and the entire body feels energized and healthy.

Basic Breathing Techniques

The first two techniques I will be teaching you are the basic breathing techniques, which can be used on their own or combined with the postures, relaxation or meditation techniques. The most important part to remember is that if you are sitting your spine should be as straight as possible and the chest open. If the shoulders are hunched forward, the breathing is constricted and the upper spine curved. In order to straighten the spine further, pull up through the crown of the head so that the back of neck lengthens and you can feel the lengthening of the entire spine. Imagine an invisible string attached to the crown of your head pulling you up. Also be aware of sitting downward on each buttock, to ground you. This two-way action up and down will create the poise you need in the body for all the benefits of the breath to take place.

While practising your breathing, try to be aware of how your body feels. Which parts of the body are rising and falling or expanding and contracting? Perhaps even take your hands to the areas you are focusing on and watch your hands go up and down, or move apart and come together. Feel the breath passing through the nostrils with each inhalation and exhalation. Begin to understand the effect every breath is having on the body and mind.

There are three main areas in the torso used in breathing. The first area is the abdomen: it brings air into the deepest and lowest parts of the lungs. Abdominal breathing is slow and deep, and the diaphragm is properly used.

Intercostal breathing, or middle breathing, is the second area and involves the rib muscles expanding the ribcage.

Clavicular breathing is the third area. During inhalation, the shoulders and collarbone are raised while the abdomen is drawing in a little.

Before you start the techniques below, take a few minutes to focus on each of these areas, inhaling and exhaling slowly and deeply, so that you can become familiar with how each feels in your body.

Abdominal Breathing

Abdominal breathing is best done lying flat on the ground in Corpse Pose (savasana: see page 30).

1. Place one hand on the abdomen. The ideal spot is over the belly button.
2. Now take a deep, slow breath, using as much of the lower part of your abdomen as possible. As you inhale, feel the abdomen rising and expanding into your hand, and as you exhale, feel the abdomen falling. Really feel your hand rise and fall as you breathe. Don't look at your abdomen – keep your head flat on the ground, and try to feel the motion.
3. Continue this for a minute or so.

Initially it might seem strange to be using the abdomen, and your breathing might feel tired and unnatural. This is fine, and all part of learning. Gradually you will start to breathe like this all the time. You may even struggle to remember how you used to breathe. This is common as well, and seeing students discovering how to breathe properly again is always a great pleasure.

Awareness: Physical – on the quality of breath, relaxing the body, and the rise and fall of the abdomen. Energetic – on manipura chakra.

Full Yogic Breath

The full yogic breath, which can be practised both sitting or lying in Corpse Pose, occurs through three stages. First, the abdomen expands through the process of abdominal breathing. Then you inhale sideways into the ribcage, using the intercostal muscles to expand the ribcage and draw the air into the middle part of the lungs. Lastly, air is inhaled into the upper part of the chest: clavicular breathing. You will notice that the three types of breathing spoken about on the previous page – abdominal, intercostal and clavicular – are all incorporated into the full yogic breath in order to gain the maximum benefits from each inhalation and exhalation.

1. Lie on the ground in Corpse Pose (savasana) or sit comfortably cross-legged. Place cushions under the buttocks if needed. The important thing is to be relaxed and comfortable, with the spine as straight as possible. If the back is uncomfortable, try sitting against a wall.
2. Place one hand on the abdomen and the other on the chest to feel them rising and falling as you breathe.
3. Inhale slowly and deeply, feeling the abdomen expand as you inhale. Once the abdomen is reasonably full, continue to inhale through the ribcage and finally feel the air filling the upper chest and shoulders.
4. Pause for a moment and experience your lungs being full, then begin your exhalation, letting all the breath out of the body until none is left, leaving a feeling of

emptiness with no strain at the bottom, simply quiet. Pause for a moment, enjoy the stillness and quiet, and wait for the in-breath to arrive once more. And so the journey of breath continues.

5. Feel each part of the body expand and contract as you inhale and exhale. Always be relaxed, keeping your breathing at a steady flowing pace, and stay completely aware of the breath, pausing at the bottom and top of each one. It is so easy for the mind to wander off, and you won't experience the true benefits if you don't completely absorb yourself within the breath.

Awareness: Physical – on the quality of breathing, relaxing the body and feeling the various parts of the abdomen, ribs and chest rise and fall. Energetic – on manipura or anahata chakra.

Pranayama

Pranayama is the Sanskrit name for more advanced breathing techniques. It translates as 'restraint' or 'control of the vital force'. These techniques should be attempted only once you are completely familiar with the basic breathing techniques above.

All of these techniques should be practised in a seated position. You may choose any of the sitting positions which are discussed in more detail on pages 166-7, in the chapter on meditation. In the instructions overleaf I will assume you are already sitting comfortably in the pose of your choice.

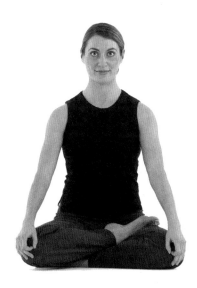

Ujjayi Breathing (Victorious Breath)

Ujjayi Breathing helps to create internal heat and energy in the body. The Sanskrit word *ujjayi* derives from the root *ji*, which means 'to conquer', and the prefix *ud*, which means 'bondage'. It is the breathing technique that gives freedom from bondage and is said to liberate one from disease.

1. Begin by breathing deeply through the nostrils. Concentrate only on the inhalation and exhalation.
2. As your awareness becomes attached to the breathing, transfer your focus from the nostrils to the throat. Now imagine that your breath is being drawn into and out of the throat, as if there is a small hole there.
3. As the breathing becomes slower and deeper release the chin into the chest slightly, which closes the glottis. (The glottis is the flap of skin that helps stop food going down the windpipe.) This produces a gentle hissing or snoring sound, which should be smooth and steady as you breathe.
4. Both inhalation and exhalation should be long, deep and controlled.
5. Practise full yogic breathing while you concentrate on the sound in the throat produced by the breath. The sound shouldn't be too loud. It should only be loud enough to be heard by another person if they are sitting close to you.
6. Continue for up to 10 minutes – beginners may want to do short sittings until comfortable with the technique.

Advanced variation

As you become more comfortable in Ujjayi Breathing, begin to bring in a retention of the breath (for however long is comfortable but without strain) between the inhalation and exhalation. Be aware of the pause between the breaths and enjoy the stillness that it brings. This retention is known in yoga as *kumbhaka*.

> **Benefits:** Ujjayi Breathing, with its concentration on the hissing sound during inhalation and exhalation, is a meditative breath. The quality of the sound should tell you about your own mental state at that moment. It has a profoundly relaxing effect on a psychic level. It soothes the nervous system and calms the mind. It can help to cure insomnia. It slows down the heartbeat and is useful for people suffering from high blood pressure.

> **Contraindications:** Pregnant women should not retain the breath during the practice of any pranayama techniques.

> **Awareness:** Physical – on the throat, the sound of the breathing and the lengthening of the breath. Energetic – on vishuddhi chakra.

Alternate Nostril Breathing

Have you ever noticed that you are generally able to breathe more easily through one nostril than the other? Or that you are completely blocked on one side, and then, a little while later, it is the other nostril that is blocked? The breath alternates between the right and left nostril about every 90 minutes in a healthy person. If you are unable to breathe through one nostril for over two hours it is considered to be a sign that illness is imminent. Alternate nostril breathing balances both nostrils and energy flow in the body.

I will discuss two forms of alternate nostril breathing. Both use the same hand positions. Take your left hand and place it on the left knee. Take your right hand and fold the index and middle finger down to the palm of the hand so that the thumb and two end fingers are straight. Or make a fist and then open out the thumb and two end fingers. This hand position is called 'vishnu mudra'. Maintain this hand position throughout. In both techniques close the eyes and relax the body.

Alternate Nostril Breathing Without Retention (Nadi Shodhana)

Take a deep, slow inhalation and exhalation. Close the right nostril with the right thumb.

1. Inhale through the left nostril a smooth and steady breath.
2. When you have completed a full inhalation, close the left nostril with your ring finger. Remove the thumb to open the right nostril.
3. Exhale through the right nostril a smooth and steady breath.
4. When you have a completed a full exhalation, inhale through the right nostril a smooth and steady breath.
5. When you have completed a full inhalation, close the right nostril with your thumb. Remove the ring finger to open the left nostril.
6. Exhale through the left nostril a smooth and steady breath.
7. This is one complete round. Repeat 10–12 times (or more if it feels comfortable).

Benefits: Balances the flow of breath in the right and left nostrils, as well as the right and left sides of the entire body. Calms the mind and body. Regulates the breathing tempo.

Common mistakes: The inhalations and exhalations are of different duration. Try to focus on making the breaths equal length on both sides.

Awareness: Physical – on the rhythm and quality of the breath. Energetic – ajna chakra.

Alternate Nostril Breathing With Retention (Anuloma Viloma)

This form of alternate nostril breathing brings retention of the breath, kumbhaka, into the sequence and also begins to control the inhalation and exhalation to specific counts. The general ratio for the inhalation–retention–exhalation is 1–4–2. In the beginning try using counts of 4 for the inhalation, 16 for the retention and 8 for the exhalation. If the retention of the breath is at all uncomfortable for this duration, don't worry about bringing it down to a count of 12, for instance. The goal, however, should be eventually to hold for 16. Of course, as you develop your technique, you can begin to experiment with higher counts, such as 8–32–16, or even higher. Just remember to keep that 1–4–2 ratio in the technique. As before, begin in the basic sitting pose with the right hand in vishnu mudra ready to block the nostrils. Take a deep, slow inhalation and exhalation.

1. Block the right nostril with the right thumb. Inhale through the left nostril to a count of 4.
2. Block both nostrils gently with the thumb and ring finger. Retain the breath for a count of 16.
3. Release the thumb from the right nostril. Exhale through the right nostril to a count of 8.
4. Inhale through the right nostril to a count of 4.
5. Block both nostrils gently with the thumb and ring finger. Retain the breath for a count of 16.
6. Release the ring finger from the left nostril. Exhale through the left nostril to a count of 8.
7. This is one complete round. Repeat 10–12 times.

As with the first alternate nostril breathing technique, feel free to do more than 10 or 12 rounds if you feel the benefits from this. There is no maximum number of rounds, just as there is no maximum count for the inhalation–retention–exhalation, although 27–108–54 is considered auspicious, highly energetic and beneficial, among ancient yoga texts!

Benefits: Balances the left and right sides of the breathing as well as of the body. Extra oxygen is taken into the body and the brain centre is stimulated, leading to clearer thinking and increased mental activity. Vitality is increased and stress and anxiety are lowered.

Common mistakes: Rushing through your counting. Try using a counting metre to control the count, for instance: 'Om 1, Om 2, Om 3, Om 4,' and so on. This helps you keep the rhythm to your breath and also keeps the mind focused on the technique.

Awareness: Physical – during inhalation and exhalation, on smooth and steady breathing; during retention, on relaxation of the body. Energetic – During inhalation and exhalation, on the chakra of your choice. During retention, on ajna chakra.

Pumping Breath (Kapalbhati)

Kapalbhati is literally translated as 'shining skull', because of the cleansing benefits associated with it. The pumping breath involves a vigorous drawing in of the abdomen during exhalation. The pumping action should be practised before starting – if you do not have the correct action, the rest of the technique loses a lot of its effectiveness.

The pumping action: sitting comfortably, put your hands on your abdomen so you can feel it moving during inhalation and exhalation. Once you feel comfortable with the pumping action then place your hands on the knees for the technique. Inhale and feel the abdomen expanding. Exhale forcefully, squeezing the abdomen back as far as you can and then repeat this action: inhale abdomen expands, exhale forcefully squeezing abdomen back as far as you can. Keep this action going until it feels comfortable in your body. To help, visualize a plastic bottle full of water. Picture squeezing the middle of the bottle tightly so that water shoots out of the top. This is what you are trying to achieve with the pumping action: squeezing your abdomen and forcing the air to shoot up and out of the nostrils. Gradually the exhalation should be the dominant breath, with the inhalation just being an automatic reaction after the exhalation. When you are comfortable with that, then you are ready to begin the full technique.

1. Close your eyes and keep them closed. Inhale and exhale two full yogic breaths.
2. Inhale and expand the abdomen, and on the exhalation, begin the pumping breath. Continue at a steady and comfortable pace for a count of 30 pumps.
3. Exhale completely at the end of the final pump. Inhale and exhale two full yogic breaths.
4. Inhale to three-quarters capacity and retain the breath for up to 30 seconds.
5. Exhale slowly and deeply.
6. This is one complete round. Repeat for at least three complete rounds

The number of pumps and the length of retention given above are guidelines. Once you feel comfortable in the technique, begin to add on additional pumps (for example, 10 per round) and retain the breath for longer periods (for example, 30, 45 then 60 seconds – though never 'for as long as I can'. Always state a specific target for pumps and retention before you start).

Benefits: Purifies the bloodstream and removes excess carbon dioxide from the body. Revitalizes the body and clears the mind. Removes excess phlegm from the system and clears the bronchial passages. Removes drowsiness and lethargy. Tones the abdomen and helps concentration. Tones the digestive organs. Balances and strengthens the nervous system.

Common mistakes: Getting the pumping breath wrong! (Practise the action before starting.) Rushing the technique. (It is the quality not quantity that counts.)

Contraindications: Pregnant women should not practise kapalbhati.

Awareness: Physical – during pumping, on the motion of the abdomen; during retention, on relaxation. Energetic – during pumping on manipura chakra; during retention on ajna chakra.

Cooling Breath (Sitali)

This is a great technique to use after a long session of any physical activity because it cools the system down. It is one of the few times in yoga practice that you breathe through the mouth. Begin in your normal sitting pose with both hands on the knees.
1. Close the eyes and relax the body.
2. Extend the tongue outside the mouth as far as possible.
3. Roll the sides of the tongue up so that it forms a tube. If you can't roll your tongue, keep it flat, place the tip of it on your lower lip, and try to touch the middle of the tongue to the roof of the mouth for support.
4. Inhale and draw the breath in through this tube (or over a flat tongue as described above). You will hear a sound like rushing wind and feel a cool sensation.
5. At the end of the inhalation, draw the tongue in and unroll it. Close the mouth.
6. Exhale through the nose.
7. The inhalations and exhalations should be long and full yogic breaths. This is one round. Repeat 10–12 times, or as much as is comfortable. In hot weather do as many as you please.

Benefits: Cools the body and mind. Affects important brain centres associated with temperature control. Encourages free flow of energy through the body. Gives control over hunger and thirst. Helps reduce blood pressure and stomach acid.

Contraindications: Those with asthma or low blood pressure should not practise sitali.

Awareness: Physical – on smooth and steady inhalations and exhalations. On the sound of the inhalation and the cooling sensation of the breath. Energetic – on vishuddhi chakra

Relaxation

By letting go, it all gets done.

Tao Te Ching

The act of relaxation is central to yoga. Learning to relax properly is every bit as important as learning to perform the postures correctly. In yoga the postures are used to create additional energy for our system. Proper relaxation seals this energy, cares for it and provides a space for it to flow through our entire being. As you spend more and more time in proper relaxation, you will begin to become aware of just how tense you previously were, and what true relaxation feels like. If the postures are tools to energize and invigorate, then proper relaxation is a tool to cool down and balance the system.

Every physical action creates tension in our muscles. We often experience this tension, whether it is because of extreme physical exertion, or a result of a long day sitting at a desk in front of a computer, the back curled forward and the shoulders hunched. Most of us have come to accept this tension as a natural part of our lives, may even have convinced ourselves that we perform our daily routines better in a state of tension, as if tightness and strain assist, rather than hinder, our efforts. This is not the case. Any performer or athlete will confirm that at their best, an unconscious relaxation of the body naturally takes place, allowing them to perform their job efficiently and to the best of their abilities. Proper relaxation is a gift every one of us should give to our bodies each and every day.

The mind can be just as tense as the body. Uncontrolled emotion uses up as much energy as physical activity, although we are seldom aware of this. Proper relaxation is about letting go of emotions, observing them for what they are, and understanding their changing and impermanent nature.

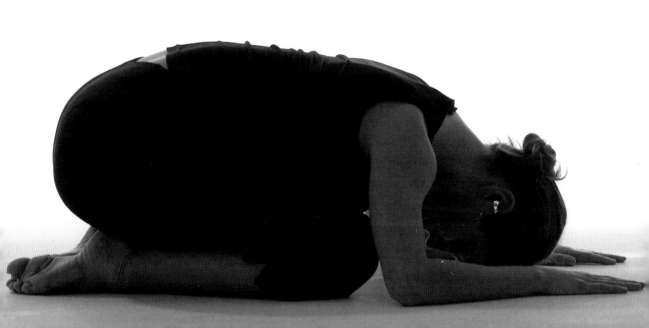

Corpse Pose (Savasana)

Corpse Pose requires you to lie flat on the ground, completely relaxed, and simply breathe. Relaxation before, during and after any physical exercise is vital in order to bring your heartbeat back to normal, circulate fresh air and energy (prana) through your body, eliminate lactic acid (which causes tiredness and is produced when exercising) from your muscles and relax you mentally.

1. Lie down flat on the ground, with eyes closed and your chin tucked slightly towards your chest, lengthening the back of the neck. Keep the head still.
2. Straighten your legs and move them about hip-width apart with the toes relaxed and falling out to the sides.
3. Place your arms flat and away from the body, proba-bly at about a 45-degree angle, and turn your palms up. Relax your arms, fingers and shoulders.
4. Think about your entire spine relaxing towards the ground. Your lower back might be slightly raised from the ground. This is normal.
5. Focus on breathing naturally through the nose, being aware of how it feels to breathe in this position.

Variation

For anyone with a bad back who finds lying flat with straight legs uncomfortable, try bending the knees and placing the soles of the feet flat on the ground. This relieves pressure on the lower back.

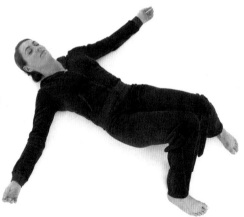

> **Awareness:** Physical – on the breathing, relaxing the body. Energetic – on the chakra of your choice.

Child's Pose

This relaxation can be done at any time during your pratice. Begin by sitting on your heels. Slowly take your forehead to the ground in front of you. When the forehead touches the ground, place the arms alongside the body reaching behind you, palms up, elbows and shoulders relaxed. Close the eyes. If this is not comfortable try parting the knees slightly or placing a pillow under the forehead. Or make a pillow with your hands and rest the head on that. Breathe normally and visualize relaxation moving through the body.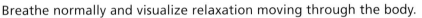

Awareness: Physical – on the breathing, relaxing the body. Energetic – on the chakra of your choice.

Lying on Front

This relaxation pose should be done between backbending postures, such as Cobra, Locust and Bow.

1. Lying flat on your abdomen, bend the elbows and make a pillow with your hands by placing the hands on top of one another, palms down, directly under the head.
2. Separate the legs hip-width apart, with the toes turning in towards each other. This opens the lower back. Place one cheek on the pillow, looking to one side, and relax the entire body.
3. Close the eyes and breathe normally.

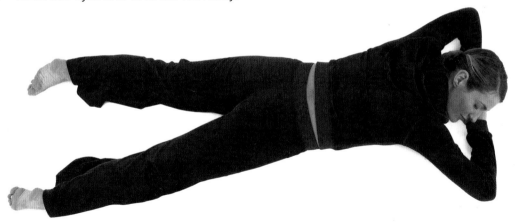

Awareness: Physical – on the breathing, relaxing the body. Energetic – on the chakra of your choice.

Initial Relaxation

To be done before any postures.

Lie flat in Corpse Pose (savasana) and be aware of your breathing. How does it feel? Mentally check every part of your body. Are there any aches and pains that could hinder your yoga practice? If so, imagine your breath sending energy directly to those parts of your body that are feeling tense or uncomfortable. Constantly return to the breathing and allow it to relax your body and mind. Inhale energy through your body, exhale tension with each breath. Let go of worries. Relax and give the next twenty minutes, or half an hour, or however long you wish to practise, to yourself. This is your time, so make the most of it. Stay in this position for a few minutes until you feel fully relaxed.

Relaxation Between Postures

After each posture use the breath to return to a state of deep relaxation and examine what effect the posture has had on your body. Your breath may be hurried and your muscles tense after some of the postures, so use this time to balance the energy in the body and return to a comfortable state. Do not begin the next posture until your breath has returned to normal and your body feels relaxed and energized by fresh intake of oxygen and energy.

Final Relaxation

Too many of us finish any type of physical exercise without properly bringing the body and mind back to a relaxed and comfortable state. We carry on with our day without allowing the full benefits of our practice to sink in and circulate through the body. Final relaxation is vital and at least 5 minutes (ideally 15 if you were practising for an hour or more) is necessary to scan your body and mind and ensure that you have relaxed every part of it. There are two main types of relaxation: physical and mental. Each brings its own benefits, and they should be practised one after another slowly and with full awareness of the breath at all times.

Physical Relaxation

Since it is often hard initially for beginners to relax, it is important to understand what it feels like for the body to be tense as well. Understanding tension often allows the beginner to relax further than they thought possible. Try it and see. Lie in Corpse Pose (savasana) and breathe steadily. You are gradually going to tense and relax various parts of the body; always remember to breathe through the nose and be aware what your body is telling you. Remember as a rule to inhale to tense and exhale to release.

- Inhale and raise the right leg 5cm (2 inches) from the ground. Tense the entire leg, feel the tightness right through the leg. After 3–5 seconds of tensing, exhale and relax the leg and allow it to drop to the ground by itself. If dropping your leg like this is uncomfortable, you may have lifted your leg higher than 5cm from the ground. Repeat the above with your left leg.

- Inhale and raise the hips 5cm from the ground, pressing down through your heels and lifting the groin area upward. Tense the buttocks and backs of the legs. Hold the tension for 3–5 seconds and then exhale and relax completely and allow the hips to fall back to the ground.
- Inhale and lift the chest off the ground. Tense the upper body and feel the shoulder blades coming closer together behind your back. Hold for 3–5 seconds, then relax and gently drop the chest to the ground.
- Inhale and raise the right arm 5cm from the ground. Tense the entire arm. Hold for 3–5 seconds. Now clench your fist, then extend your fingers as much as possible. Exhale, release and let the arm fall gently to the ground.
- Repeat with the left hand.
- Lift the shoulders towards the ears, inhale and tense.
- Drop the shoulders towards your feet, exhale and relax.
- Inhale and scrunch your entire face. Tense every part of your jaw, cheeks, eyes, ears and forehead. Imagine you have just eaten a lemon!
- Tilt your head slightly back, open your eyes and mouth as wide as possible, let your tongue hang out (try to touch your chin with it) and silently let out a large exhalation.
- Now just relax and be aware of how the entire body feels. Take a few moments to check each part, creating a mental checklist that you can go through each time you relax.

Mental Relaxation

After tensing and relaxing each part of the body, you are ready to use auto-suggestion to deepen your state of relaxation. Take your time with this one. The mind has a habit of wandering and at first it might be hard to concentrate, especially knowing the technique is almost over.

- Feel as though a wave of relaxation is sweeping over your entire body and then down to your toes. Use the breath to imagine clean air and energy coming into your body with every inhalation. On the exhalation, concentrate on releasing negative energy or physical blockages. Beginning with the toes, mentally relax each one, telling yourself slowly as you breathe out, 'I am relaxing my toes, I am relaxing my toes, my toes are relaxed.' As you go through, repeat this relaxation command for each part of your body, focusing on the part and feeling it relax.
- Now proceed to your feet and ankles. Feel the relaxation sweeping through these parts of your body. Take as much time as you need. Feel the difference. Always use the exhalation to tell your body to relax. Inhale energy, exhale tension.
- Exhale and feel the relaxation moving up the legs, relaxing the calves, the knees, the thighs. Repeat the relaxation command for each part individually and be aware of how each part feels as tension is gradually released.
- Exhale and relax the buttocks and feel the tension releasing from your lower back. Take time to concentrate on the back. This is very important. Your back is under so much strain throughout the day: give it this moment to relax properly. Feel the lower back begin to sink towards the ground.

- Feel the relaxation proceeding to your chest, breathing very slowly and gently.
- Now bring your attention to the fingers and on an exhalation keep repeating the relaxation command to yourself, quietly and patiently, always using the breathing to pace yourself.
- Slowly come up through the wrists, arms, elbows, shoulders. The shoulders are another place to focus your attention closely. As with the lower back, feel the shoulders relaxing into the ground. You should feel as though you would drop through to the centre of the earth if the floor weren't there to stop you.
- Exhale and relax the neck, jaw, chin, cheeks, mouth, eyes and forehead. Imagine your entire face melting, especially the cheeks, eyes and jaw. The face holds an enormous amount of nervous tension and you should feel this tension disappearing. Just relax and observe how your body feels right now. Take a few moments to rest in this position and make time in your life just to be.

Note: This book is not directed at women who are pregnant. However, there is no reason why pregnancy should affect your relaxation technique in any way. See what is comfortable for you. If lying flat on your back is uncomfortable, bend your knees and definitely after 30 weeks turn sideways so that you are lying on your left-hand side, with your right palm flat next to your head as if you were going to sleep. Do what your body tells you – always.

Sun Salutation

With hands in prayer I face the sun, feeling love and joy in my heart.
I reach out and let the sun fill me with warmth.
I bow before the sun's radiance and place my face to the ground in
*   humble respect.*
I lift my face to the sun and remember, to achieve such heights I must be
*   as the dust of the Earth.*
I stretch up towards its light trying to reach the greatest heights, and again
*   surrender.*
I stand tall as I remember the true sun is within me.

The Sun Salutation is a great way to begin or end any day. In fact, it can be done any time (except after eating), it stretches just about any part of the body you want and it has been a part of yoga for thousands of years. A long time ago the sun was worshipped as a god, bringing light and heat to everything. People must have thought the Sun Salutation was pretty special to name it after the most powerful thing in their world. It is special, and even done by itself can bring huge benefits to anyone.

The Sun Salutation is a sequence of movements that should be done in time with the breathing. For every inhalation there is an up or forward movement, and for every exhalation there is a down or backwards movement. Initially you should not worry too much about the breathing. Concentrate instead on getting each movement correct, especially how to move from one posture to another. This is the part that often causes problems for beginners. Take your time and get comfortable in each posture. Sometimes it helps to begin by breaking down the postures into threes and practising small parts, so that the movements between each posture are properly understood. In time the breathing will naturally flow on top of the movement.

It is important that you don't go too quickly. Think about letting your body move at a steady pace throughout, so that the same amount of time is spent in each posture. Always think about relaxing any part of the body that may be tight, and as you go along be aware of how different muscles are stretching. The correct speed for you is probably the speed of a good deep breath. Since each posture (except one) is done on an alternating inhalation and exhalation, then you shouldn't be moving more quickly than your breathing.

As you become more comfortable with the movements, you should start to think about the three basic elements of the Sun Salutation: the physical postures, the breathing process and the mental attitude.

The Physical Postures

There are twelve postures in the Sun Salutation. Twelve is the number of the zodiac and the number of months in a year. Understand the way that the postures join together and turn into one continuous movement. Try to flow through the sequence without thinking of each posture as an individual one. It is all part of the entire movement. Like a dance!

The Breathing Process

Work towards breathing in perfect rhythm with the movements of the body. Bring the breathing in tune with the body. As the breathing relaxes the body, the movements will become easier and the enjoyment will increase. Take proper deep inhalations and be sure to exhale fully each time, but with no strain.

The Mental Attitude

Be focused and aware of how both the body and the breathing are functioning. Keep the thoughts directed towards what you are doing right now, and be aware of every change as it occurs. As this awareness grows, you will suddenly discover that your breathing, body and mind are working together, in union. Eventually, when you are comfortable with the flow of movements with the breath, you can add the mantras to your practice. They can be repeated out loud but it may be easier to say them silently so you can also include the breath within your practice.

Benefits

The Sun Salutation is said to strengthen and tone up to 140 different muscles. Loosens and invigorates the body. Stretches, massages, tones and stimulates all the muscles, vital organs and physical parts by alternately flexing the body backwards and forward. Sun Salutation is a complete sadhana, spiritual practice, in itself, as it comprises posture, breathing and, for advanced students comfortable in the technique, the possibility also to include mantra and meditation.

Common mistakes

Not flowing from one posture to another smoothly and not combining breath with movement. Study the individual postures used in this sequence and be sure that your technique is correct.

Contraindications

None

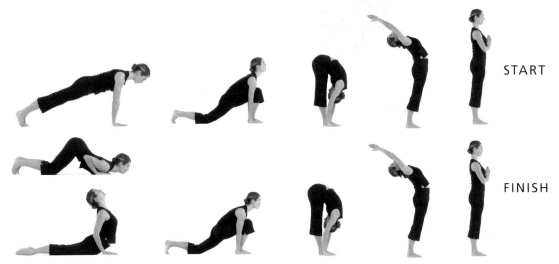

START

FINISH

Sun Salutation (Surya Namaskar)

1. Stand in Mountain Pose (tadasana). Inhale and take the arms sideways, stretching them out and up.

   Awareness: Physical – on coordinating breathing with flowing movement. Energetic – on anahata chakra.
   Mantra: Om mitraya Namaha (om mit-ri-a na-ma-ha)

   Exhale and bring the arms down and into prayer position, palms together in the middle of your chest. Maintain the lift through your waist, feeling the abdomen firm as well.

2. Inhale and take the arms straight up in front of the face, stretch them all the way up so that the palms are facing each other and the arms are reaching for the sky. Feel the spine stretch and lengthen. Tilt the pubic bone forward and up slightly.

   Begin to go backwards from the hips. Reach up with the hands throughout. Bend backwards as far as you are comfortable. If the breathing is restricted in any way then you have gone too far. Don't tip the head back too far; try to keep the neck in line with the arms.

   Awareness: Physical – on coordinating breathing with flowing movement. Energetic – on vishuddhi chakra.

   Mantra: Om ravaye Namaha (Om ra-vi-ay na-ma-ha).

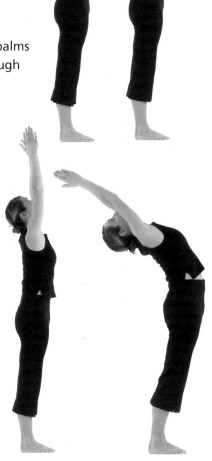

3. Exhale and bend forward from the hips into a Standing Forward Bend. Continue to fold over and try to place your hands by your feet, tops of the fingers and toes in line (twenty in line) and palms pressed into the ground either side of the feet. If you are able to place your hands flat then you should keep them in this exact spot throughout the sequence. If your hands don't reach the ground, then bend the knees to assist you. If you bend the knees, remember to keep pressing up through the tailbone in order to stretch the hamstring muscles.

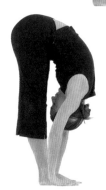

Awareness: Physical – on coordinating breathing with flowing movement. Energetic – on swadhisthana chakra.
Mantra: Om suryaya Namaha (om sir-yi-ay na-ma-ha).

4. On a deep inhalation, press down through the hands and lift the right foot. Now take a large step back with the right leg, as far as you can go. Allow the right knee to release to the ground. Bring your head up and look straight ahead. Press your shoulders down and back, feeling your chest open. The palms of your hands should be flat on the ground. Sink down through the pelvis, feeling the stretch in the buttocks, thighs and hamstrings.

4. Variation

When you step back the leg, it is also an option to keep it straight with the knee off the ground, pressing back through the heel. (This can also be done in step 9.)

Awareness: Physical – on coordinating breathing with flowing movement. Energetic – on ajna chakra.

Mantra: Om bhanave Namaha (om ba-na-vay na-ma-ha).

5. Retain the breath, press down through the palms and lift the left foot and take the left leg back to meet the right. You should now be in the Plank Pose. Hands and arms should be directly under the shoulders, head and neck in line with the spine. You should be looking down at the floor just in front of you. Keep the abdomen and legs firm. Press the heels back and down into the ground in order to straighten the body.

5. Variation

Instead of retaining the breath and stepping back into Plank, there is an alternative movement that I like both to do and to teach, which you can try as well. From step 4, step back the left foot on an exhalation and press back into Inverted V (Downward Dog), hold for a brief moment, then on an inhalation lower the hips and bring the head forward into Plank. You will now be in the same position as above with the breathing ready to continue into step 6.

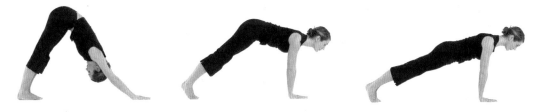

Awareness: Physical – on coordinating breathing with flowing movement. Energetic – on vishuddhi chakra.

Mantra: Om khagaya Namaha (om ka-guy-a na-ma-ha).

6. Before exhaling, bring your knees down to the floor. If it is more comfortable turn your toes back so that the tops of your feet are flat on the floor. Push your hips and buttocks slightly backwards. Your hands should still be under your shoulders, and your knees under your hips.

    Now exhale and bring the chest and chin to the floor. Push back through the hips while you release the downward pressure through the palms so that your buttocks seem to rise in the air as your chest falls between your hands. Try to make sure you keep your hands in the same position throughout. Check that your elbows are tucked into the body and the shoulders are relaxed.

    Awareness: Physical – on coordinating breathing with flowing movement. Energetic – on manipura chakra.

    Mantra: Om pushne Namaha (om push-nay na-ma-ha).

7. Inhale and glide the upper body forward and between the hands and move into Cobra. Keep your shoulders down and back, and remember to keep your elbows tucked in. The feet are pointed.

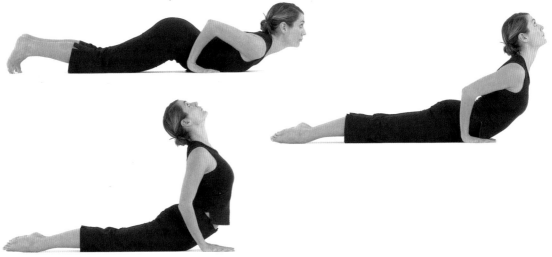

    Awareness: Physical – on coordinating breathing with flowing movement. Energetic – on swadhisthana chakra.

    Mantra: Om hiranyagarbhaya Namaha (om hear-an-ya-gar-bia na-ma-ha).

8. Exhale, tuck the toes underneath, press down through the palms to straighten the arms, push the tailbone back and up, and lift the buttocks up to the sky into Inverted V. Try to make the movement into Cobra, then out of Cobra and into Inverted V smooth and steady. This is one to practise just by itself. The movement should be similar to a seesaw action.

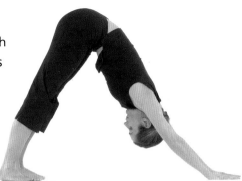

Awareness: Physical – on coordinating breathing with flowing movement. Energetic – on vishuddhi chakra.

Mantra: Om marichaye Namaha (om ma-rich-aye-ay na-ma-ha).

9. Inhale and bring the weight forward through the arms, and lift the right foot and step it forward between the hands. The left knee should drop to the ground as you step and inhale.

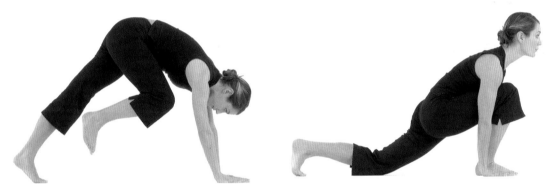

If you find this step too much at present, take the leg as far forward as possible, then help it along by taking hold of the ankle and lifting it between the hands. This movement will loosen up in time – just keep practising.The head should also now come up and you should feel a sink down through your buttocks.

Variation
It is also an option to keep the leg straight with the knee off the ground, pressing back through the heel. (This can also be done in step 4.)

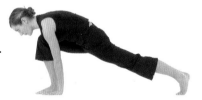

Awareness: Physical – on coordinating breathing with flowing movement. Energetic – on ajna chakra.

Mantra: Om adityaya Namaha (om ad-it-ya-ay na-ma-ha).

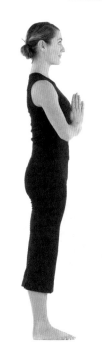

10. Exhale, press down through the right foot, push gently forward through the left foot and come back to standing, with the body folded as far down over the legs as possible, in a Standing Forward Bend. The fingers and toes of both sides should be in line on the ground with palms pressing down. If you need to, bend your knees.

    Awareness: Physical – on coordinating breathing with flowing movement. Energetic – on swadhisthana chakra.

    Mantra: Om savitre Namaha (om sa-vi-tray na-ma-ha).

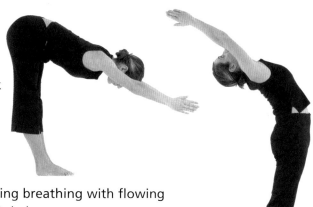

11. Inhale and reach forward and up with the hands. Allow your arms to lead the rest of your body up. Keep the neck extended and keep the back lengthened. Go back all the way up to standing. If comfortable, tilt the pubic bone forward and up and slightly reach back as in step 2.

    Awareness: Physical – on coordinating breathing with flowing movement. Energetic – on vishuddhi chakra.

    Mantra: Om arkaya Namaha (om ark-aye-a na-ma-ha).

12. Exhale and return to prayer position, palms together in front of the chest.

    Awareness: Physical – on coordinating breathing with flowing movement. Energetic – on anahata chakra.

    Mantra: Om bhaskaraya Namaha (om bas-car-ray-a na-ma-ha).

Repeat the whole sequence using the left leg to go back and come forward first. After finishing both the right and left sides you have completed one full round. Begin by doing a few rounds and gradually build up to six or nine at a time, possibly adding one round a week.

Standing Postures

Life is practise, practise is life.
Judith Lasater

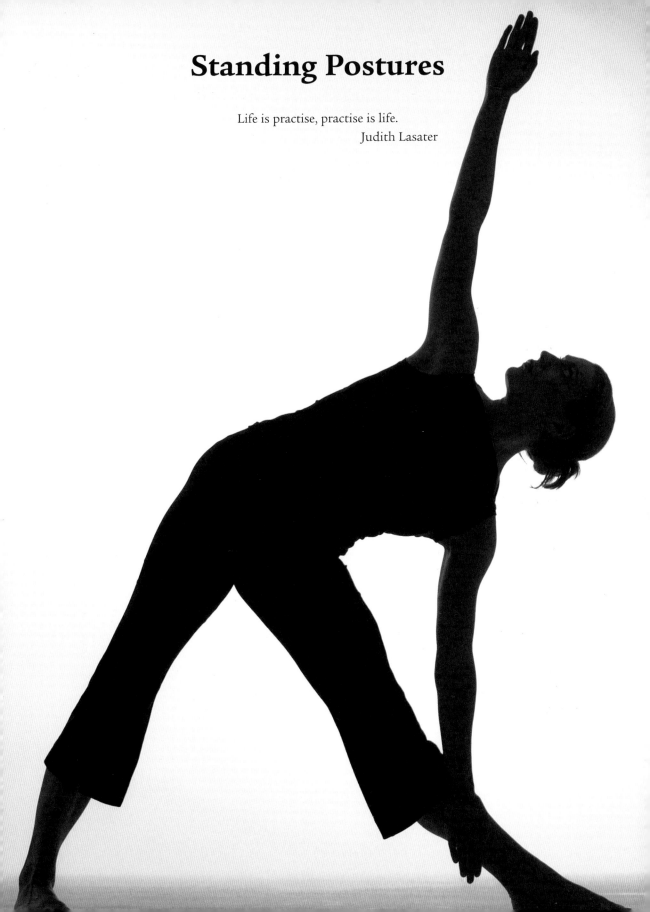

Standing postures are some of my favourite poses: they heat and stimulate the body and help develop balance and stability. They are usually practised at the beginning of a session after the Sun Salutation to prepare the body well for the following postures.

Mountain Pose (Tadasana)
Level: 1

How often do you stand up straight and tall during your daily life instead of leaning to the left or right, or slouching forward? Proper posture is vital to yoga, and nowhere is that more important than when standing up straight on two feet. The Mountain Pose is an active posture; it isn't as simple as just standing. Ample time should be spent in the Mountain Pose in order to feel the body erect and tall, as strong as a mountain.

1. Stand tall with the feet together, the heels and big toes just touching each other. Feel the heels and balls of the feet pressing down equally into the ground, providing a firm foundation for the body. Maintain an even distribution of weight on the feet throughout. Stretch the toes out and plant them firmly onto the ground. Imagine your feet pushing roots into the ground just as a mighty tree would, giving balance and strength.

2. Tighten the thighs slightly so that the kneecaps lift, but don't lock them. Squeeze the buttocks to tilt the hip and tailbone down and forward slightly.

3. Lift the chest up and lengthen the back of the neck, keeping the chin parallel to the ground. Feel the elongation of the spine as your upper body pulls away from the waist.

4. Imagine an invisible string attached to the crown of your head pulling you upward. Relax your shoulders and allow them to drop, creating distance between the ears and shoulders.

5. Allow your arms to fall evenly down by the side of the thighs, neither ahead of nor behind the body.

In the proper Mountain Pose you should feel as if your upper body is pulling in the opposite direction to your lower body, creating length in the spine. Your balance may initially feel wobbly in the proper standing posture; this will obviously change in time with practice. Eventually Mountain Pose will be regarded by your body as the easiest and most comfortable standing position.

Tree Pose (Vrksasana)
Level: 1

The Tree Pose is the first of the 'basic' balancing postures in the standing sequence. As the name suggests, this posture is all about feeling as if you were a tree establishing roots in the earth to provide balance and coordination. Just as the wind blows a tree from side to side without toppling it, so in Tree Pose you might feel your balance wavering from side to side. Experiment, and don't get frustrated if your balance is better on one side or the other – this is normal for beginners. If your balance is really wobbly, use the wall as a support.

Start in Mountain Pose (tadasana).

1. Find a fixed point to focus on directly in front of you. Maintain this point of focus throughout.
2. Shift your entire weight onto the left foot by lifting the heel of the right foot. Ensure you are properly balanced before proceeding. Ensure that the left leg is active by tightening the thigh and buttock and lifting up through the waist.
3. Bend your right leg and place the right heel on the side of the left calf, or, if you are comfortable, on the side of the thigh. You may use your hands to assist this movement. Rest the foot down onto the inside of the leg so that the toes point down. Anywhere is fine, just so long as the foot does not press against the side of the knee joint.
4. Once your balance is secure, bring the palms of your hands together in front of your heart in prayer position. Feel free to stay in this position, focusing on the breath. However, to advance the posture, slowly stretch your arms straight above your head, palms together. Stay in the pose for a few seconds, breathing normally.
5. After remaining in the posture for a few seconds, slowly lower the arms, maintaining balance. Straighten the right leg and relax in Mountain Pose (tadasana).
6. Repeat the posture on the other leg, trying to remain balanced for an equal length of time on both sides.

45

Advanced variation

1. From Mountain Pose (tadasana), bend your right leg and lift the heel onto the top of the thigh in Half Lotus, so that the top of your foot is pressing into the thigh just below the groin area. Push the right knee back and away, ensuring the left hip does not swing forward. It is vital to keep the tailbone dropping downward.

2. Once your balance is secure, take your hands into prayer position and then slowly stretch your arms straight above your head, palms together. Stay in the pose for a few seconds, breathing normally. Slowly lower the arms, maintaining balance. Straighten the right leg and relax in Mountain Pose (tadasana).

3. Repeat the pose on the other leg, trying to remain balanced for an equal length of time on both sides.

4. As your balance improves you may extend the length of time spent in Tree Pose to a maximum of one minute on either side. When you are fully comfortable in the pose you may want to try closing your eyes and keeping your balance, but be ready to tumble!

Benefits: The Tree tones the leg and buttock muscles and gives a sense of balance and poise. The side muscles of the torso are toned and stretched when the arms are raised. Concentration is enhanced. Equilibrium between left and right sides is achieved.

Common mistakes: Attention is allowed to wander away from the point of focus, leading to loss of balance. Feet are in an incorrect position to begin with. Ensure that the feet are parallel, pointing ahead, not turned out.

Contraindications: None.

Sequence: During any practice of standing postures.

Awareness: Physical – on balance. Energetic – on anahata chakra.

Eagle (Garudasana)

Level: 2

The Eagle is the second of the 'basic' balancing postures in the standing sequence. Although it looks difficult, once the basic technique is mastered the actual balancing becomes easy because of the downward pressure placed on the standing foot by the rest of the body. As with the Tree, it is vital that you find a good point of focus and keep your concentration on that point. Start in Mountain Pose (tadasana).

1. Move your weight onto the left leg by lifting the right heel off the ground. Bend the left knee.
2. Bring the right leg over the left thigh above the knee making sure that there is no gap between the legs. Move the right foot behind the left calf and hook the toes around the inner side of the standing leg. If you are unable to hook the toes, don't worry – it's quite normal to begin with.
3. Find your balance in this position before proceeding. It sometimes helps to adjust the angle of bend in the standing knee, higher or lower. Also feel free to use a wall to assist your balance to begin with.
4. Bend the elbows and raise the arms to the level of the chest. Rest the left elbow on the right upper arm near the elbow joint. Now move the right arm to the right and the left to the left. The right arm will now be entwined around the left arm. Join the palms and lift the elbows to shoulder height so that your arms move away from the body at a right angle. Pull up through the fingers and straighten the spine. (If you have trouble with this arm position, perhaps give it a try on its own without the legs.) Remain in this position for up to 30 seconds with normal breathing.
5. Release the arms and legs and return to Mountain Pose (tadasana).
6. Repeat on the other side, with the left leg moving over the right leg, and the right elbow being placed above the left elbow.

Benefits: The Eagle strengthens, loosens and tones the ankles. It helps prevent cramp in the legs and improves circulation. Stiffness in the shoulders is removed. Balance and concentration are improved.

Common mistakes: The most common mistake is leaning forward in the pose. Although advanced versions of the Eagle do call for an extreme forward bend, many people find slightly bending the upper body forward makes the posture easier. This should be avoided. Don't get frustrated if you fall out of the posture: comfort in any balancing posture comes with time and practice.

Contraindications: If you have had any knee problems, approach with caution.

Sequence: During any practice of standing postures.

Awareness: Physical – on keeping your balance while concentrating on a fixed point. Energetic – on mooladhara chakra.

Fierce Pose (Utkatasana)

Level: 1

Imagine you are sitting down to help visualize yourself in this pose. However, keep the heart lifting to the sky.

Start in Mountain Pose (tadasana).

1. Stretch the arms straight out above the head and join the palms.
2. Exhale and slowly bend the knees, allowing the torso to lower as if you were going to sit down. The knees and buttocks gently squeeze together. If possible, continue to bend the knees until your thighs are parallel to the ground. Do not stoop forward. Keep lifting your chest as much as possible and keep your gaze directly forward.
3. Remain in the pose for up to 30 seconds.

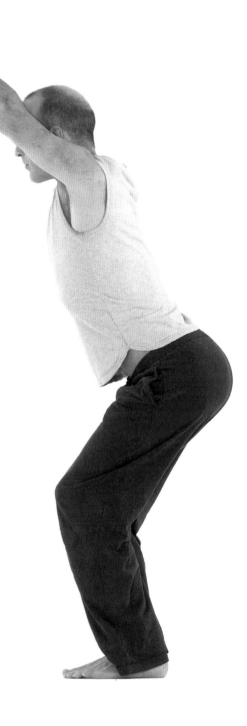

Advanced variation

Keeping your knees bent and glued together, twist your torso
to the right, lower your arms into prayer pose and
place the left elbow to the outside of the right thigh,
just above the knee. Open your chest by rotating the
right shoulder up and back. With your palms together in
prayer position, the right elbow is pointing directly up and
there is a straight line from one elbow to the other. Look up and
continue to rotate the torso, pressing the left elbow into the right
thigh for additional leverage. The rotation should be in the upper
body only, the knees and hips should remain square throughout.
Inhale, simultaneously straighten the legs slowly and lower the
arms. Relax in Mountain Pose (tadasana).

Benefits: This pose removes stiffness in the shoulders and corrects minor problems
in the legs. The ankles are strengthened and the leg muscles develop evenly. The
back is toned and the chest is developed through proper expansion. This posture is
good for those who ski.

Common mistakes: The arms are allowed to fall forward and become passive. The
head drops forward and eyes gaze straight down. Uneven weight distribution
through the feet means the body falls forward. The pelvis should stay square to the
front otherwise the alignment is incorrect.

Contraindications: None.

Sequence: During any practice of standing postures.

Awareness: Physical – on strength in the legs and lifting of the heart. Energetic –
on anahata chakra.

The Warrior Sequence

The three postures representing the Warrior sequence are some of the most beneficial and powerful of all Yogic postures. Although the first two may look fairly easy, they require great strength and concentration to hold for long periods. The third Warrior posture is an intense combination of balance, strength and awareness of the body. Combined they help build a powerful base for the body to move forward into all other yoga postures.

Warrior I (Virabhadrasana I)
Level: 1

Start in Mountain Pose (tadasana).

1. Jump or step the feet approximately 1.25 metres (4 feet) apart (not so far as to be uncomfortable in any way) and turn the right foot out 90 degrees. Turn the left heel away from you slightly. Ensure that there is a straight line from the heel of the right foot back to the heel of the left foot.

2. Turn the upper half of the body so that you are facing square in the direction of the right foot.

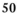

3. Bend the right knee, attempting to make the thigh parallel to the ground. A right angle should be formed between the shin and the ground. The knee should not be ahead of the ankle, but in line with the heel. Stretch out the left leg and press down through the outside of the left foot drawing up through the inner thigh. By doing this the leg muscles are engaged. This is vital for the pose.

4. Inhale and lift the arms straight above the head, in line with the ears, palms facing each other. Remember to keep breathing. The face, chest and right knee should all point straight ahead. The gaze should be up towards the hands but if this isn't comfortable you can look forward. Lift up through the head so that the spine straightens and the tailbone drops.

5. Hold the position for 20–30 seconds with normal breathing. When finished, straighten the right leg and lower the arms. Repeat on the other side.

Benefits: Breathing is improved through the opening of the chest. Stiffness in the shoulders and back is relieved and the ankles and knees are toned. The abdominal muscles and organs are toned. Fat around the hips is reduced. The legs are strengthened.

Common mistakes: The torso must be turned completely round so that it faces the direction of the front foot. Do not allow the arms to drop but keep pulling up through the fingers and elbows to extend through the waist and spine. Do not allow the weight through the back leg to ease – the back leg provides the support for Warrior so keep the pressure down through the outside of the back foot.

Contraindications: None.

Sequence: During any practice of standing postures.

Awareness: Physical – on lifting up out of the waist and arms and pressing down through the outside of the back foot. Energetic – on anahata chakra.

Warrior II (Virabhadrasana II)
Level: 1

Start in Mountain Pose (tadasana).

1. Jump or step the feet approximately 1.25 metres (4 feet) apart (not so far as to be uncomfortable in any way) and turn the right foot out 90 degrees. Turn the left heel away from you slightly. Ensure that there is a straight line from the heel of the right foot back to the heel of the left foot.

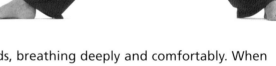

2. Lift the arms so that they are parallel with the ground, palms facing down. The arms should feel as if they are an extension of the chest, pulling away from the body and reaching in opposite directions.

3. Exhale and bend the right knee so that the thigh is close to parallel with the ground and the shin forms a right angle with the ground. The bent knee should not extend beyond the ankle. Look along the right arm towards the hand. The torso should remain facing forward, not towards either leg. Stretch out the hands as though you are being pulled in opposite directions. Maintain weight down through the outside of the left leg and foot, stretching it fully and drawing up through the inner thigh.

4. Remain in the posture for 20–30 seconds, breathing deeply and comfortably. When finished, straighten the right leg and lower the arms. Repeat on the other side.

Benefits: Warrior II shapes and strengthens the leg and shoulder muscles. Cramp is relieved in the calf and thigh muscles and the abdominal muscles and organs are toned. The body gets great elasticity through the practice of Warrior and prepares you for all other standing postures.

Common mistakes: The arms will want to drop, especially the back arm. Keep the arms strong and parallel with the ground. Do not take the front knee beyond 90 degrees with the floor. Keep pulling up the torso so that extension of the spine is achieved.

Contraindications: None.

Sequence: During any practice of standing postures.

Awareness: Physical – keeping strength and stillness in the posture.
Energetic – on mooladhara and manipura chakra.

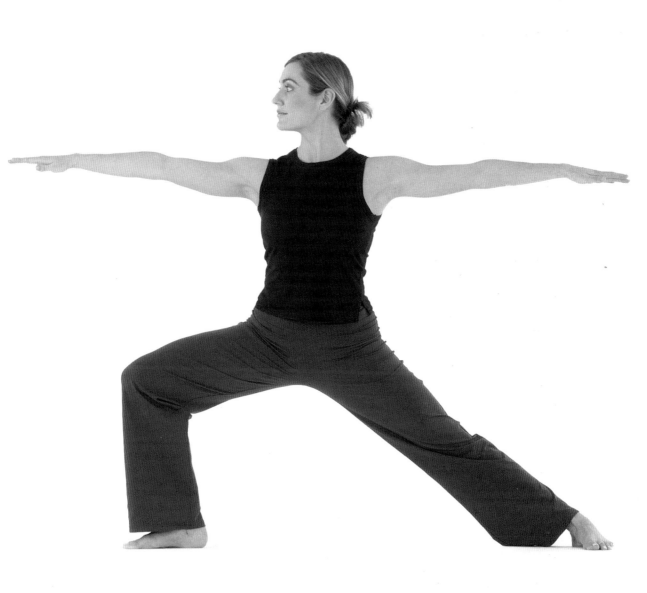

Warrior III (Virabhadrasana III)
Level: 2

Start in Mountain Pose (tadasana).

1. Turn the body to the right and bring the arms above the head, palms together. Step the right foot forward about 15cm (6 inches) and place the right heel onto the ground.

2. Begin to move the weight of the entire body forward onto the right foot only, lifting the left leg behind you as you move forward, keeping the arms in line with the ears and the body as straight as possible. Visualize your body as a pendulum, so that as your upper body moves forward and down, the back leg moves backwards and up.

3. Keep moving forward so that you are balancing only on the right leg. The entire body, from the fingertips to the left toes, is parallel with the ground. Stretch the body as if someone is pulling your hands forward and your left foot backwards. Visualize your body as a capital letter T.

4. Remain in this posture for 20–30 seconds, breathing deeply and comfortably. To come out of the posture, lower the left leg to the ground and straighten up the torso. Repeat using the other leg.

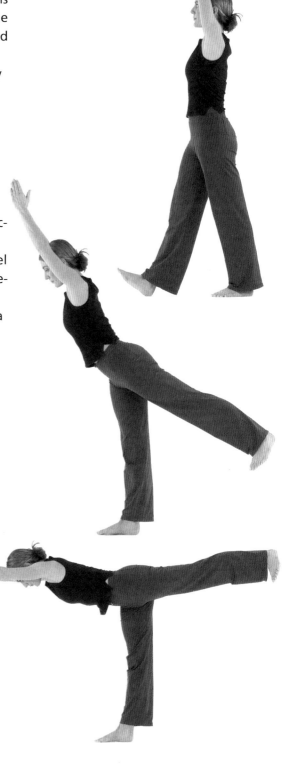

Beginner's variation

Beginners who do not feel that their balance and strength are sufficient to remain in the Warrior III for any period of time should use blocks for assistance.

1. Turn the body to the right. Place two blocks on the ground, lengthways up, approximately 30cm (12 inches) in front of you, in line with each shoulder.
2. Bring the arms above the head, palms together. Step the right foot forward about 15cm (6 inches) and place the right heel onto the ground.
3. Begin to move the weight of the entire body forward onto the right foot only, lifting the left leg as you move forward and keeping the arms in line with the ears and the body as straight as possible. Visualize your body as a pendulum, so that as your upper body moves forward and down, the back leg moves backwards and up.
4. As you extend forward and continue lifting the left leg, reach the arms down and place the hands on each block, palms down. Press down through the blocks as you continue to lift the left leg behind you up and away.
5. When your body is parallel to the ground, hold the position and breathe normally for 20–30 seconds. To deepen this stretch and as preparation for Warrior III without blocks, occasionally try to lift the left leg beyond the parallel point.
6. In order to come out of the posture, push off against the blocks and lower the left leg to the ground. Relax in Mountain Pose (tadasana), for a few seconds, and then repeat on the other side.

Benefits: Warrior III develops harmony, grace and balance in the body. It contracts and tones the abdominal organs and muscles and strengthens the standing leg. It is highly recommended for runners. Warrior III helps us to have proper technique in normal standing with the weight bearing down through the soles of the feet.

Common mistakes: Bending either leg in Warrior III is incorrect, but especially so for the standing leg, which should be kept strong and firm by engaging the thigh muscles. Keep extension running throughout the entire body from front to back, as this will assist in the balance. Keep the head still and focus on a fixed point.

Contraindications: None.

Sequence: During any practice of standing postures.

Awareness: Physical – on balance and extension of the body. Energetic – on manipura chakra.

Triangle (Trikonasana)
Level: 1

The triangle is the first lateral (sideways) bend of the spine I will be teaching. The spine is the body's central column for health and well-being. It is important to be able to bend the spine in all directions in order to keep it healthy and flexible.

Start in Mountain Pose (tadasana)

1. From standing, step or jump your feet approximately 1 metre (3 feet) apart. Turn your right foot out 90 degrees. Turn the left heel away from you slightly. Ensure that there is a straight line from the heel of the right foot back to the heel of the left foot. Maintain the pressure down through the legs without locking either knee. Raise the arms sideways, parallel to the ground with the palms facing down. Ensure that the arms remain in line with the shoulders.

2. On an exhale, lift up out of the waist and reach as far as you can towards the right-hand side, keeping the hips square, facing straight ahead. When you can reach no further, pull back slightly from the extension and keep the body in the correct alignment with the weight evenly distributed through the legs and the arms still parallel to the ground.

3. Inhale, then exhale, turn the palms forward and allow your right arm to extend down towards the right ankle, still keeping the hips square. The right hand, depending on your flexibility, will rest on your right thigh, calf, ankle, or even flat on the floor. Reach your left hand directly up towards the sky, palm facing forward, pulling through the fingertips in order to intensify the stretch down the left-hand side of the body. There should be a perfectly straight line from fingertips to fingertips. To help alleviate pressure in the right knee joint, press down on the balls and toes of the right foot.

Variation

To intensify the pose, slowly bring the left arm down so that it is in line with the ears and look up towards the armpit. Keep the left arm straight and continue to pull out through the fingertips. Work the left hip back and the right hip forward, while maintaining even balance through the legs. For support you may want to gently place your right hand on your shin.

4. Maintain the pose for up to a minute, breathing normally and continuing to square the hips and pull away through the left fingers. Visualize strings attached to the end of the fingers pulling up and away from your shoulder. The right arm is largely passive during the triangle, used mainly for balance and direction.

Advanced variation
In order to open the chest further take your left arm and place it behind the back so that your left hand touches the right thigh. Look up and turn your left shoulder up and back, feeling the chest expand as the ribcage rotates. Visualize the heart lifting up and back.

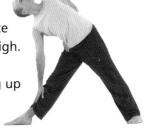

5. To come out of the posture, inhale and lead with your left fingers and arm back to the starting position, slowly straightening out the body, maintaining balance and not allowing the knees to lock. Repeat on the other side.

    Benefits: This posture tones and removes stiffness in the legs and hips. It strengthens the ankles and gives an intense stretch to the entire length of the torso. Regular practice will reduce the waistline. The Triangle stimulates the nervous system and alleviates nervous depression. It strengthens the pelvic area and tones the reproductive organs. It maintains equilibrium between both sides of the body.

    Common mistakes: The most common mistake is not keeping the hips square to the front and attempting to place the hand lower on the leg than is necessary. It is much more important to keep the hips square than it is to place the hand on your ankle or the ground. Legs should remain straight throughout. Do not allow the upper arm to become passive during the posture – it is the upper arm that controls the intensity of the torso stretch. Do not allow the body to fall forward, but keep opening the chest up and back. To test if your hips and body are square or not, you should be able to do this pose against a wall, with your heels, buttocks, upper back and hands all in contact with the wall.

    Contraindications: Those suffering from severe diagnosed back conditions shouldn't practise this posture.

    Sequence: During any practice of standing postures.

    Awareness: Physical – on coordination of movement, balance and using the upper arm to intensify the stretch down the side of the torso. Energetic – on manipura chakra.

Reverse Triangle (Parivrtta Trikonasana)
Level: 1–2

Start in Mountain Pose (tadasana).

1. From standing, step or jump your feet approximately 1 metre (3 feet) apart. Turn your right foot out 90 degrees. Turn the left heel away from you slightly. Ensure that there is a straight line from the heel of the right foot back to the heel of the left foot. Maintain the pressure down through the legs without locking back into either knee. Raise the arms sideways, parallel to the ground with the palms facing down. Ensure that the arms remain in line with the shoulders.

2. Inhale and rotate the torso so that you are facing in the direction of the right foot. Bring your left arm forward and take your right arm back, still shoulder height.

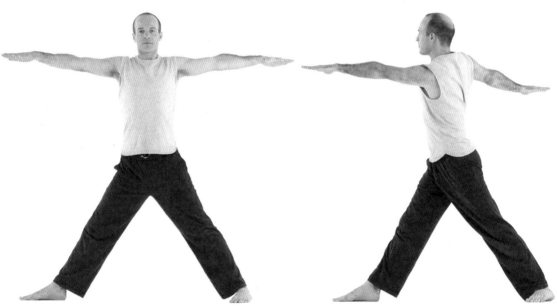

3. Exhale and reach forward taking the left hand down to the right side of the right leg or foot, placing the hand on the ground on the outside of the right foot, or pressing against the outside of the right leg, wherever is most comfortable. If you need to use a block for this posture, place the block on the right side of the right foot and then place the left hand flat on the block.

4. Stretch the right arm up, palm facing away from you, bringing it in line with the left arm. Gaze up at the right hand.

5. Continue to rotate the trunk towards the right, opening the chest and trying to lift further through the right arm. Hold the posture for 10 deep breaths.

6. To come out of the posture, drop the right arm and, inhaling, swing the left arm back up, lifting your torso as the arm swings back and up. Return to Mountain Pose (tadasana) and breathe normally, relaxing the body.

7. Repeat on the opposite side.

Benefits: The Reverse Triangle tones the thigh, calf and hamstring muscles, creating flexibility and strength in the legs. The chest is expanded fully, allowing deeper breathing. The posture increases the blood supply to the lower part of the spinal area, helping the spine and muscles of the back to function properly. It invigorates the abdominal muscles and strengthens the hip muscles.

Common mistakes: The legs should be kept straight throughout, although the knees should not lock. The upper arm shouldn't be passive, but should be lifting up throughout, stretching the shoulders. The spine should be lengthened and rotated. Weight should remain as evenly distributed through the feet as possible.

Contraindications: As for Triangle.

Sequence: Twisting standing poses are always preceded by their classical counterpart ie Triangle before Reverse Triangle.

Awareness: Physical – on coordination of movement, balance and using the upper arm to intensify the stretch down the side of the torso. Energetic – on manipura chakra.

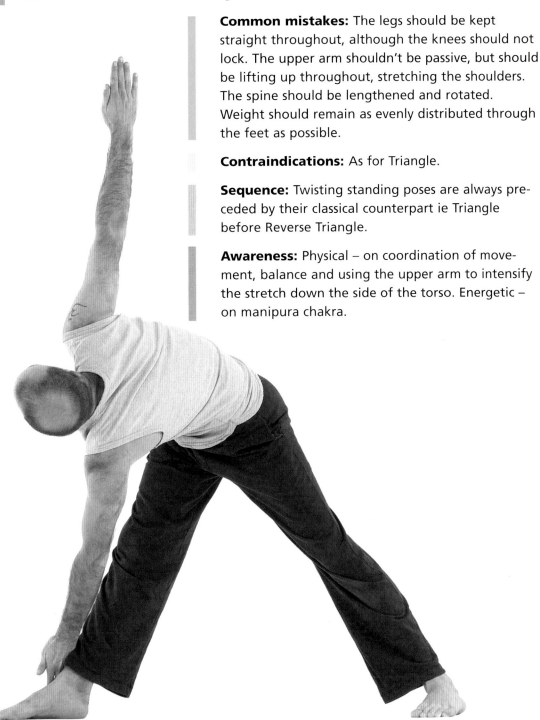

Standing Forward Bend (Uttanasana)
Level: 1

The Standing Forward Bend is one of the foundation postures in yoga, and the basis for all the standing poses. A wonderful posture, it can look easy to copy, but students often focus more on reaching the ground than on which parts of the body are being stretched. More than anything, the Standing Forward Bend is an intense stretch of the hamstrings and other leg muscles. However, it also is a spinal stretch. Carefully read the instructions for this posture below and focus on awareness of the body as you practise.

Start in Mountain Pose (tadasana).

1. Step the feet hip-width apart (hip-width is where your hip bones are, not the outside of your legs) and parallel. Inhale and reach the arms out to the side and then above the head, palms facing each other. Stretch up through the fingertips so that you can feel the muscles down both sides of the body elongating. Imagine the top half of your body pulling away from the waist and the feet grounding you.

2. Exhale and leading with the arms extend forward by bending at the hips. Keep reaching forward through the fingers as you descend. The spine should be kept straight, and as the body passes through the halfway point the spine should be parallel to the ground and not slouched at all.

3. Keep bending from the hips until you can bend no further. Only at this point relax and let the head and arms drop naturally. You should feel the hamstrings stretching. If you can touch the floor comfortably then lift up through the tailbone and try to take the head to the knees.

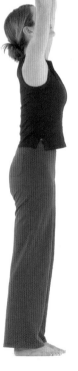
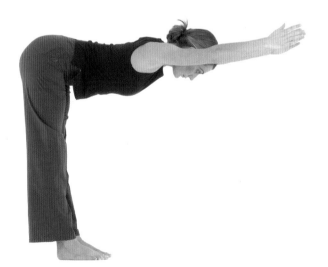
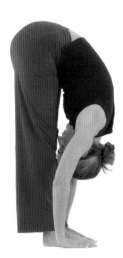

4. Remain in this pose for up to a minute, breathing deeply. Try to use the breath to take you deeper into the posture. For each inhalation imagine that your breath is opening and extending the spine and that the head is reaching out and away (visualize a weight attached to the crown of the head pulling it away – not necessarily down, that depends on your flexibility). For each exhalation relax the entire body deeper into the posture.

5. When you are ready to come out of the posture, inhale and stretch your arms forwards and up, going through the flat back pose until you are standing. Exhale, arms out to the sides and down. Or you could bend the knees slightly and roll up vertebra by vertebra using an exhalation. Visualize your spine being stacked one vertebra at a time as you unfold the body, keeping the arms and neck relaxed until your spine is completely straight. Only then straighten the neck and take the shoulders back into a standing posture. Relax and breathe comfortably.

Variations

Many students ask where their hands should be in the final position of the Standing Forward Bend. There are many answers to this question, I will highlight seven prominent variations for forward bend.

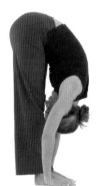

A. Palms flat on the ground: This is the 'classical' posture and also the most difficult for most beginning, and even some intermediate, students. It involves placing the palms flat on the ground either side of the feet, with the tips of the fingers in line with the tips of the toes. If you can achieve this, great. If not, don't worry, as you can get great benefits from the posture without being able to move into this pose.

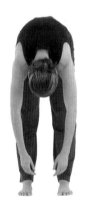

B. Rag doll: Perhaps the most popular position for most beginners. Just relax the entire body and allow the arms to hang freely to whatever point you are comfortable. Keep the legs engaged, as described above.

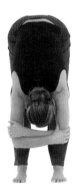

C. Holding the elbows: When you have descended into the final position, take hold of each elbow with the opposite hand. The extra weight this produces should intensify the stretch and allow you to move slightly deeper into the pose.

D. Big toes: If you are able to, take hold of the big toe of each foot with your index and middle finger, palms facing in towards each other on an exhalation. Try to pull yourself just a little deeper into the stretch by allowing your elbows to bend outwards, but keep the shoulders relaxed away from the ears.

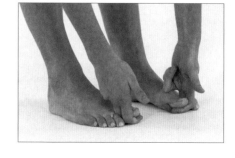

E. Hands under the feet: If you able to, place the fingers, or even the entire hand, under each foot with the palms facing up, and step down onto the fingers. You should feel it down the hamstrings the moment you step down as the new angle of the ankle bend created by the hands under the feet stretches the hamstrings further. Try to take more weight onto your hands as you become more familiar with the pose.

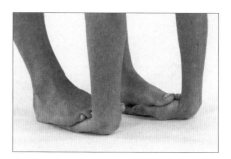

F Holding the ankles: For those with limited flexibility who find all the above quite difficult, you can also simply hold onto the legs as far down as you can go. Whether that is the ankles or the shins is fine.

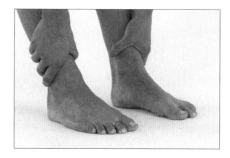

G. Hands interlocked behind: Take the arms behind you and try to interlock the hands together. Then lift the arms as far as you can. Once again, this should intensify the stretch by increasing the downward pressure of the torso. This movement also should lift the tailbone, lengthening the hamstrings further.

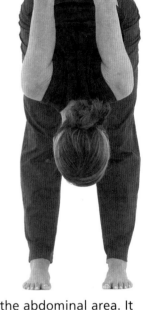

Benefits: The Standing Forward Bend reduces excess fat in the abdominal area. It improves digestion and blood circulation in general due to the inversion of the upper body. It strengthens the legs and tones the leg muscles. It improves balance and general flexibility.

Common mistakes: The most common mistake is to slouch forward into the bend, allowing the spine to curve. Although this may initially allow you to drop further, in the long run it will limit your progression. Maintain a straight spine as you descend, feeling the hamstrings engage as you go down. Only when you reach a point where you can bend no further from the hips should you allow the spine to curve at all. Remain active in the posture throughout; do not allow yourself to simply go to sleep in the bend. Keep awareness throughout the body and use the breathing continually to take you further into the bend. Keep the back of the neck relaxed. Make sure that the weight is evenly distributed across the feet, not swinging back onto the heels.

Contraindications: None.

Sequence: During any practice of standing postures.

Awareness: Physical – on the pelvic area, using the breath to deepen the stretch. Energetic – on swadhisthana chakra.

Wide-leg Forward Bend (Prasarita Padottanasana)
Level: 1

The Wide-leg Forward Bend uses the same upper-body principles as the Standing Forward Bend, with the obvious difference that this time the legs are separated to a comfortable degree, bringing the stretch into the inner thighs and outer calves, as well as the hamstrings.

Start in Mountain Pose (tadasana).

1. Jump or step the feet approximately 1 metre (2–3 feet) apart. The feet should be pointed forward in parallel and the spine erect. Lift up through the crown of the head and feel the tailbone dropping into the space created by the wide legs.
2. Inhale and lift the arms to the side and above the head, palms facing each other. Stretch up through the fingers, creating a stretch down both sides of the torso. Visualize your upper body pulling away from the waist and press down firmly through your feet to ground you.
3. Exhale and, leading with the arms, begin to bend from the hips forward and down. Keep the spine straight and lengthened so that as your upper body passes through 90 degrees it is parallel with the ground from the waist to the tips of the fingers. As you go down keep the weight evenly distributed across the feet.
4. Continue to fold until you can go no further, then release the arms and relax the head, neck and shoulders, allowing the arms to hang freely to the ground. If you can place the palms flat on the ground then do so.
5. Remain in this position for up to a minute, breathing normally. Use the breathing to go deeper into the posture. Continue to lengthen the spine and lift the tailbone.
6. When you are ready to come out of the posture, inhale and bring the arms forward and up, lifting the upper body with the arms and extending all the way back up to a standing position. Bring the feet together and relax in Mountain Pose (tadasana).

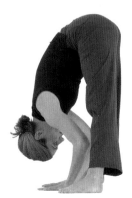

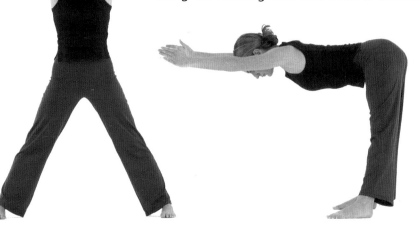

Hand variations

As with the Standing Forward Bend, there are a number of positions the hands can take in the Wide-leg Forward Bend.

A. Palms flat on the ground: Place the palms flat on the ground between the feet, with the tips of the fingers in line with the tips of the toes.

B. Rag doll: Relax the entire body and allow the arms to hang freely to whatever point you are comfortable. Keep the legs and spine active, however, as described on page 61.

C. Holding the elbows: When you have descended into the final position, take hold of each elbow with the opposite hand. The extra weight this produces should intensify the stretch and allow you to move slightly deeper into the pose.

D. Big toes: If you are able to, take hold of the big toe of each foot with your index and middle finger, palms facing in towards each other. Try to pull yourself just a little deeper into the stretch by allowing your elbows to bend outwards. Keep the shoulders relaxed and away from the ears.

E. Holding the ankles: Simply hold onto the legs as far as you can go. If that is the ankles or the shins – fine.

F. Hands interlocked behind: Take the arms behind you and try to interlock the hands together. Then lift the arms as far as you can. Once again, this should intensify the stretch by increasing the downward pressure of the torso. This movement also should lift the tailbone, lengthening the hamstrings further.

Benefits: In the Wide-leg Forward Bend the hamstring and inner-thigh muscles are fully stretched, and blood is allowed to flow to the head with the inversion of the upper body. General flexibility is increased and the legs are strengthened for all other standing postures.

Common mistakes: The most common mistake is to slouch forward into the bend, allowing the spine to curve. Although this may initially allow you to drop further into the bend, in the long run it will limit your progression. Maintain a straight spine as you descend, feeling the hamstrings engage as you go down. Only when you reach a point where you can bend no further from the hips should you allow the spine to curve at all. Remain active in the posture throughout; do not allow yourself to simply go to sleep in the bend. Keep awareness throughout the body and use the breathing continually to push you further into the bend. Keep the legs straight throughout, engaging the thighs, lifting the kneecaps. Keep the weight of the body evenly distributed across the feet, not swinging back onto the heels.

Contraindications: None.

Sequence: During any practice of standing postures.

Awareness: Physical – on the pelvic area, using the breath to deepen the stretch. Energetic – on swadhisthana chakra.

Upper Body Twist in Wide-leg Forward Bend
Level: 1–2

This advanced variation brings a spinal twist to the basic Wide-leg Forward Bend, stretching the sides of the body and further toning the abdominal area as well as strengthening the spinal column. Balance is improved and the shoulders are loosened and toned.

Variation I

This posture can also be practised using a block if you are unable to place your palm flat on the ground. In that variation simply place a block on the ground in front of you directly under your head. Then use the block to press down onto with one hand and continue with the movement.

From the Wide-leg Forward Bend place your left hand flat on the ground directly under your head. Lift the right arm to the side and above you, palm facing out. Rotate the torso as your right arm rises so that your chest opens and your gaze turns up towards the lifted hand. Try to maintain your hips square to the ground so you don't allow your pelvis to rotate. You are trying to create a straight line from the hand on the ground to the tips of your right fingers. Hold the pose for up to 30 seconds, breathing deeply and trying to keep lifting the right hand higher and rotating the torso. To come out of the posture simply lower the right hand and rotate the torso back to centre. Relax in rag-doll position for a few seconds. Repeat to the other side.

Variation II

This variation is only possible for those who can comfortably hold their ankles in the Wide-leg Forward Bend. Take the right hand and bring it across the body to take hold of the outside of the left ankle. Wrap your left arm around the back and try to rest the hand on the top of the right thigh. If your left hand is unable to do this, then simply go as far as you can and hold on to the back of your trousers. It's important to keep the hips square; don't allow your pelvis to rotate. The rotation in this pose is only in the torso. Hold the pose for up to 30 seconds, continuing to open the chest and rotate the torso. When you are ready, come out of the posture by simply rotating the torso back to centre and releasing the right hand from the left ankle. Hang in rag-doll position for a few seconds and then repeat to the other side.

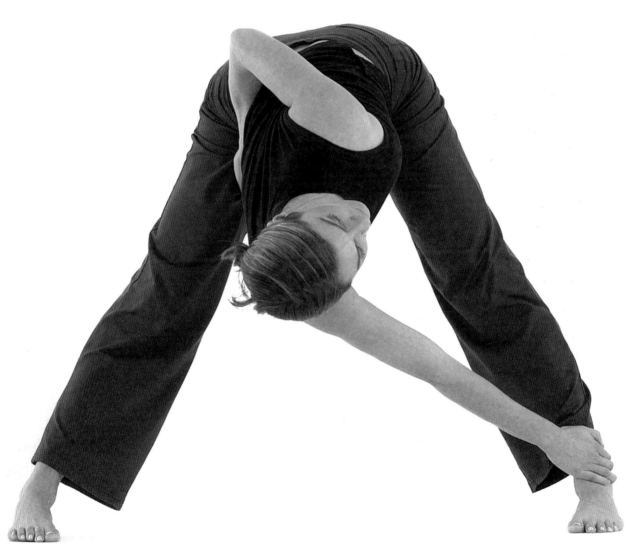

Extended Side Angle Pose (Utthita Parsvakonasana)
Level: 1–2

The Extended Side Angle Pose continues to strengthen the muscles of the legs.
Start in Mountain Pose (tadasana).

1. Jump or step the feet approximately 1–1.25 metres (3–4 feet) apart. Turn the right foot out 90 degrees and the left heel back slightly. Bend the right knee so that the thigh is parallel to the ground and the right shin forms a right angle with the ground. Rest the right elbow on the right thigh and ensure that weight is being taken back through the outside of the left foot. If the rest of the posture is too intense for your hips and legs move straight to step 4.

2. Place the right hand flat on the ground to the right side of the right foot. Lift the left hand up and try to place it alongside the ear, palm facing down, fingers reaching away from the body. The arm should be in line with the rest of the body. Look up towards the armpit, smile and breathe!

3. Try to keep extending the body into one long line. There should be weight going down through the left leg into the outside of that foot. The right arm should be extended away in line with the ear. If the arm is dropping forward due to lack of shoulder flexibility, then lift it a bit higher up in order to get it eventually in line with the ear.

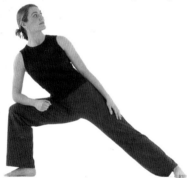 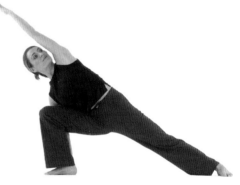

Beginner's variation
If you feel that you immediately lose your balance placing the hand on the outside of the right foot, then feel free to place the hand flat on the ground to the left side of the right foot, with the right arm pressing against the inside of the right thigh. If you are still unable to place the hand flat on the ground, then simply balance on the fingertips or a block. The left arm should be straight up in the air, palms facing forward.

4. Remain in this posture for up to 30 seconds, breathing deeply and sinking the pelvis into the pose.

5. To come out of the posture, inhale and lift the right arm and bring it back to the side of the body, then push up through the right leg to straighten the leg.

6. Relax for a few moments in a comfortable position and then repeat to the other side.

Advanced variation

This variation brings a bit of a spinal twist into the posture and further strengthens the bent leg by placing more weight on it. From the position described in step 1 above, take the left arm behind you and try to dangle it behind your back. The right arm should then come down in front of the right thigh and reach between the legs in order to hold the left hand. Once the hands are held together, rotate the torso to the left, sinking into the pelvis but remembering to keep the back leg and foot active. Remain in this position for up to 30 seconds, then release the hands and straighten the right leg. Relax for a few moments, then repeat to the other side.

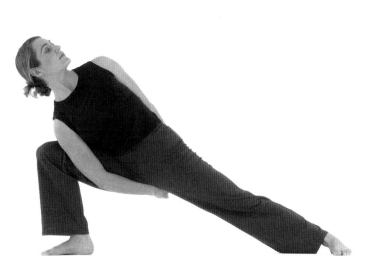 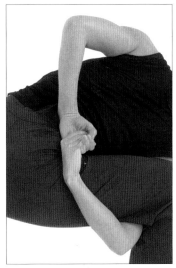

Benefits: This posture tones the ankles, knees and thighs as well as bringing looseness into the shoulders. The opening of the chest improves respiration and deepens breathing. It corrects problems in the calves and thighs and reduces excess fat around the waist. It also aids digestion.

Common mistakes: Many students will take all the weight on the front bent knee, which is harmful and can lead to knee injuries. There should always be weight back through the extended straight leg. Do not allow the raised arm to come forward or move back behind the ear. Keep it in line with the ear even if that means that it is raised away from the ear – in time the shoulder will loosen and allow the arm to release. Open the chest to assist the posture. Keep the torso opening throughout so that you can look into the armpit in the full posture.

Contraindications: None.

Sequence: During any practice of standing postures.

Awareness: Physical – on extension of the body and strength in the legs. Energetic – on manipura chakra.

Half Moon Pose (Ardha Chandrasana)
Level: 2–3

Like Warrior III, the Half Moon Pose is a challenging yet dynamic balancing posture that should first be attempted using blocks or a wall, or both, for assistance.
Start in Mountain Pose (tadasana).

1. Jump or step the feet approximately 1metre (3–4 feet) apart. Turn the right foot out 90 degrees and the left heel back slightly. Simultaneously turn to face towards the direction of the right toes and bend the right knee, placing the right hand on the ground approximately 30cm (12 inches) in front of your right toes. The right hand should be flat on the ground, fingers pointing away, but a simpler variation is to balance on the fingertips of the right hand. If you cannot reach the ground comfortably, then place a block where the hand would be and place the right hand flat on the block for assistance. Your left arm should be alongside the body.

2. Begin moving the weight forward. As more weight begins to come onto the right leg and right hand, the left foot should begin to peel from the floor, moving you onto the left toes.

3. As the left leg lifts from the ground, you should straighten the right leg. Continue lifting the left leg until it is parallel with the ground.

4. Lift the left arm straight into the air above the shoulder, palm forward. Lift up through the left arm. The ribcage should feel as if it is rotating upward to the left and the hips should be square to the front. Visualize a string attached to the top hip lifting and opening the pelvic area square to the front. The kneecap and the toes of the left leg should face forward, not upwards. Gaze up towards the left hand.

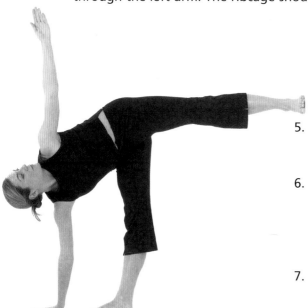

5. Hold the posture for as long as possible, breathing rhythmically. The pose should feel balanced and strong.

6. To come out of the posture bring the left arm back down alongside the body. Gently soften the right leg, bending the knee slightly, and begin lowering the left leg to the ground. Return to the starting position.

7. Relax in Mountain Pose (tadasana) for a few moments and repeat to the other side.

Beginner's variation

In addition to using a block, the use of a wall is also recommended to assist balance. Begin by standing with your back to a wall and proceed through the steps described above, just keeping the back of the body against the wall. You should find that the support the wall gives you allows you to balance far easier and open the body upward.

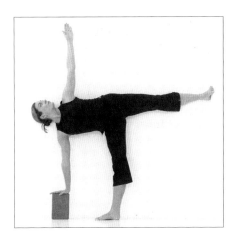

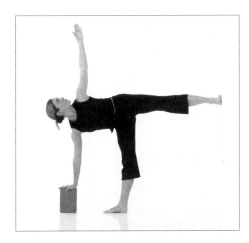

Intermediate variation

Once again use a wall with or without a block, but this time simply to press the raised foot against it. This will further assist you to feel stronger in the pose and enable you to open the chest and pelvic area to a greater degree. Simply begin the preparation for the pose by placing the supporting foot a leg length away from a wall. Follow the steps as above, then when the raised leg is parallel to the ground you should be able to press the raised foot into the wall to assist you deeper into the pose.

Benefits: The posture tones and strengthens the legs. The chest is opened, encouraging respiration. The shoulders are loosened. Balance and concentration are improved.

Common mistakes: The worst mistake would be to bend the supporting leg while in the posture. Both legs should be as straight as possible while holding the full pose. The raised arm should not be passive: use it to lift and open the front of the body. The pelvic area should be square – there is a tendency for the top hip to fall forward, so keep it moving back and up.

Contraindications: Those with knee problems should approach with caution.

Sequence: As part of a standing sequence, especially during any triangle or lunge work.

Awareness: Physical – balance and lifting up through the upper body. Energetic – on anahata chakra.

Standing Split-leg Stretch (Parsvottanasana)
Level: 2

The Standing Split-leg Stretch brings great benefits to the lengthening of the hamstrings and toning of the upper body. Once again, balance and technique are vital in this posture. Start in Mountain Pose (tadasana).

1. Step the left leg behind you about 1 metre (2–3 feet) and turn the left foot open to the left so that the sole of the foot can be firmly pressed into the ground. Adjust the space between your feet accordingly until you can find a comfortable position where the hips are facing directly forward.

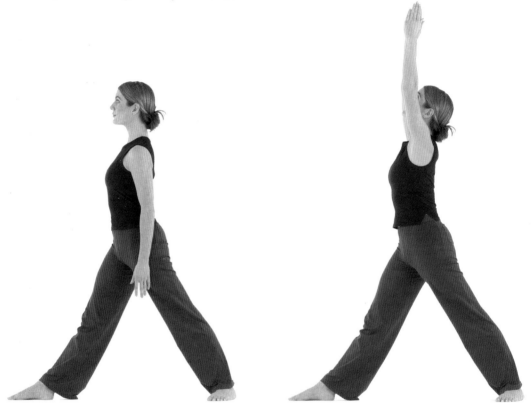

2. Inhale and lift the arms to the side and up above the head, stretching through the fingers so that you can feel the stretch down both sides of the body. Check that your legs are straight and that the hips and right foot are pointing directly forward.
3. Exhale and, leading with the arms, fold from the hips into a forward bend over the right leg. Straight away you should feel the hamstrings stretch, keeping your hips square to the front at all times. Continue to extend forward through the arms as you descend.
4. When you have folded as far as possible, allow the arms to drop to either side of your right foot. If you can rest your head on your knee, do so. Press down on the balls and toes of the right foot to alleviate pressure in the right knee.

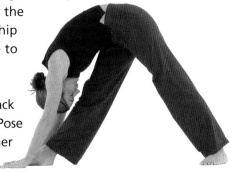

5. Remain in this posture for up to 30 seconds, breathing normally. Use the breathing to extend your spine and deepen the stretch. Keep the right hip lifting back and the left hip rotating forward, creating a square pelvis. Continue to maintain the downward pressure through the feet.

6. To come out of the posture, bend the right knee slightly and, leading with the arms, bring the body back up to the starting position. Step back into Mountain Pose and relax for a few moments. Then repeat on the other side.

Beginner's variations

It is very common for beginners to have extreme difficulties with this posture, which is why there are variations designed specifically to help them. In all of them I would recommend that you go no further down than to have your torso parallel with the ground. In doing this you can focus on extension of the spine and lengthening of the hamstrings. In time your body will tell you that you can go further. All four of the variations require you to position the body as in step 1 of the basic posture above. I will continue with the directions for each variation from that point.

A. Take your hands behind your back and take hold of each elbow with the opposite hand; now open your chest. Inhale and extend the body upward and straighten the spine. Exhale and slowly fold from the hips, extending out of the spine as you go forward and down, keeping your hips square. When you have reached a point where your torso is parallel with the ground, remain in this position, extending forward on each inhalation and relaxing the body on each exhalation.

B. Interlock your hands behind your back. Pull down and back through the arms and hands in order to open the chest and bring the shoulders back. Inhale and extend the body upward and straighten the spine. Exhale and slowly fold from the hips, extending out of the spine as you go forward and down. As you descend begin lifting the arms as high as you can behind you, pulling away through the hands and keeping the arms straight. When you have reached a point where your torso is parallel with the ground, remain in this position, extending forward on each inhalation and relaxing the body on each exhalation.

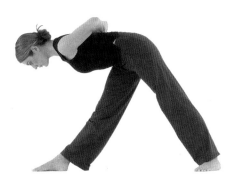

C. Allow the arms to hang down the side of the body. Lengthen through the fingers in order to feel the shoulders gently engaging. Inhale and extend the body upward and straighten the spine. Exhale and fold from the hips, extending forward all the time as you go. As you descend the arms should remain alongside the body, fingers lengthening away, chest open. When you have reached a point where your torso is parallel with the ground, remain in this position, extending forward on each inhalation and relaxing the body on each exhalation.

D. Place two blocks in front of you, one on either side of the right foot. Keep the arms alongside the body. Inhale and extend the body upward and straighten the spine. Exhale and fold from the hips, extending forward all the time as you go. As you descend the arms should remain alongside the body, fingers lengthening away, as in variation C. When you reach a point where the torso is parallel to the ground, release your arms and place the hands on top of the blocks. Press down through the blocks as you extend forward.

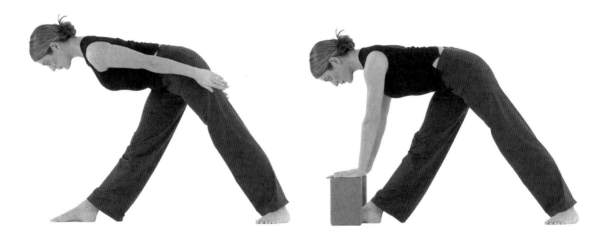

For beginners there is also the option of bending the front knee if the posture is too intense with straight legs – do remember to keep your hips square, though. Have patience and focus on awareness and technique.

Benefits: This posture relieves stiffness in the legs and hip muscles. It makes the hip joints more mobile and tones the abdominal organs. The waist is toned and excess fat removed. The posture corrects drooping shoulders and provides a firm base for all standing postures. The variations tone and strengthen the back muscles.

Common mistakes: The most common mistake occurs at the very beginning as many students do not correctly square their hips over the front leg. Many students hunch into the posture as soon as they feel the hamstrings engage; at this point it is in fact vital to achieve extension to the spine to lengthen those muscles.

Contraindications: None.

Sequence: During any practice of standing postures.

Awareness: Physical – on balance and extension of the spine. Energetic – on swadhisthana chakra.

Crescent Moon (Anjaneyasana)
Level: 1

Although this posture starts with you on your knees, it technically comes within the standing postures sequence as it can be entered with a full lunge backwards from standing or from Forward Bend. Start on your knees with your arms at your sides. Ensure that your spine is straight by pulling up through the crown of your head, feeling the spine lengthen and the tailbone drop slightly downward.

1. Inhale and step your right leg forward so that your thigh is parallel to the ground and your knee forms a 90-degree angle with the ground. Place your hands on top of the right knee. The left knee, shin and foot should be flat on the ground with your left thigh forming about a 45-degree angle with the ground. Bring the pelvis forward and down, feeling a stretch through the left thigh and groin area.

2. Maintaining the downward pressure through the pelvis and front foot, exhale and bring your hands together to prayer position in front of your heart. Maintain the length of the spine by simultaneously pulling up through the crown of the head.

3. Inhale and lift the arms above the head extending through the spine away from the waist, arching the upper back slightly and releasing the head backwards (don't drop it, though). Visualize your face lifting up to greet the sun. Lift up and back through the fingertips and down and forward through the pelvic area. The right thigh should release so that a diagonal line is formed between the left and right thighs.

4. Breathe comfortably and hold for six slow, rhythmic breaths.

5. Return to the beginning position by releasing your arms through the prayer pose and allowing the pelvis to lift and move backwards. Return your hands to your right knee. Return the right leg to the beginning position. Repeat on the left side.

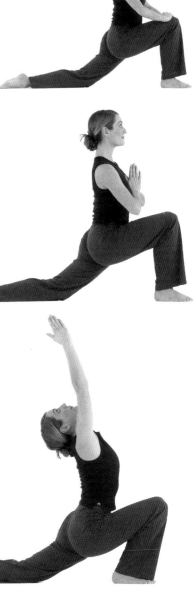

Advanced variations

Although not technically variations on the Crescent Moon, these additional postures involve the same starting position and lunge back as the Crescent Moon. The postures may be done with the back knee down on the ground, or, for more advanced students, with the knee lifted and balancing only on the balls of the back foot. Obviously the versions with raised knee are much more vigorous, so students should ensure they are comfortable with the knee down before continuing to a raised-knee version. The variations will assume that you are already in the starting position explained in Crescent Moon above.

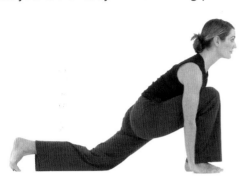 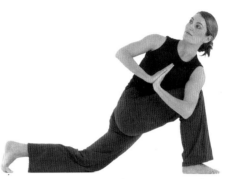

A. Step the right leg forward so that your thigh is parallel to the ground and your knee forms a 90-degree angle with the ground, and place both hands flat on the ground on either side of the right foot. Lift both hands from the ground, bring the left arm across to the outside of the right thigh and press the left upper arm into the outside of the thigh. Rotate the body open as you press. Take the right arm and raise the elbow to the sky, and bring the palms together into prayer position, trying to create a straight line from elbow to elbow and looking up and back as the chest opens and torso rotates. Try to lift and rotate the entire ribcage and abdomen over the right thigh. Hold for up to 30 seconds, breathing normally. When you are ready, release the hands, lift the left upper arm from the thigh and rotate back to starting. Step the right foot back and relax the body, perhaps in Child's Pose. Repeat to the other side. If you are comfortable with this variation then try it with knee raised. From the starting position above step forward the right leg so that your thigh is parallel to the ground and your knee forms a 90-degree angle with the ground, and place the hands to either side of the right foot. Then lift the knee and press back through the left heel, straightening the left leg. Go through the rest of the steps of this posture as explained above with the knee raised.

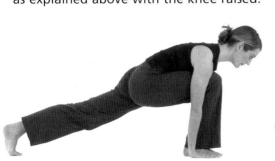

B. Step the right leg forward so that your thigh is parallel to the ground and your knee forms a 90-degree angle with the ground, and place both hands flat on the ground on either side of the right foot. Move the right hand to the side, inhale and bring the left arm straight up and then across the body. Exhale and place the left hand on the ground to the right side of the right foot so that the left arm is pressing against the outside of the right leg. (If you cannot get your hand to the floor, use a block to press down on.) Breathing steadily lift the right hand directly into the air, palm facing to the right, and look up at the extended hand. Keep extending through the raised hand. Open the chest and squeeze the left arm against the right leg to rotate the torso further. Try to lift and rotate the entire ribcage and abdomen over the right thigh. Hold this position for up to 30 seconds, breathing normally. When you are ready, lower the right hand and place it on the ground outside the left hand. Lift the left hand and return back to your start position. Step the right foot back and relax the body, perhaps in Child's Pose, for a few moments. Repeat to the other side. If you are comfortable with this variation then try it with knee raised. From the starting position above step forward the right leg so that your thigh is parallel to the ground and your knee forms a 90-degree angle with the ground, and place the hands on either side of the right foot. Then lift the left knee from the floor and press back through the left heel, straightening the left leg. Go through the rest of the steps of this posture as explained above with the knee raised.

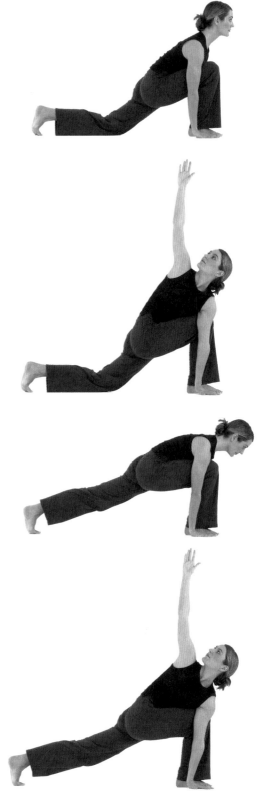

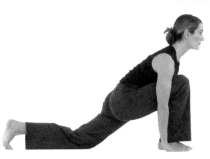 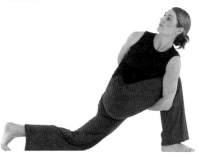

C. Step the right leg forward so that your thigh is parallel to the ground and your knee forms a 90-degree angle with the ground, and place both hands flat on the ground on either side of the right foot. Rotate the body to the right, bring the left arm across the body and try to place the left hand between the legs. The right hand should go behind the back and try to hold the left hand between the legs. Use this motion to open the chest and take the shoulders back. Try to lift and rotate the entire ribcage and abdomen over the right thigh. Hold for up to 30 seconds, breathing normally. When you are ready, release the hands, and rotate the body back to square. Step the right foot back and relax the body, perhaps in Child's Pose. Repeat to the other side. If you are comfortable with this variation then try it with knee raised. From the starting position above step forward the right leg so that your thigh is parallel to the ground and your knee forms a 90-degree angle with the ground, and place the hands on either side of the right foot. Adjust the left foot so it is as far back as possible. Then lift the left knee and press back through the left heel, straightening the left leg. Go through the rest of the steps of this posture as explained above with the knee raised.

Benefits: This pose limbers and strengthens the skeletal system, and is especially beneficial for female ailments of the ovaries, uterus and urinary tract. A full stretch of the chest and neck is obtained, relieving respiratory ailments. Balance and posture are also improved.

Common mistakes: It is important in Crescent Moon and its variations that a full stride forward is taken to begin in order to properly align the body. Do not allow the arms to become passive; it is not important how far back you can arch, but rather how well you are able to stretch the front of the body by pulling up through the arms. Do not allow your head to drop back in the final position if it causes any discomfort to the neck.

Contraindications: None.

Sequence: After forward bending postures or any practice of standing postures.

Awareness: Physical – on the lift in the upper back, on the stretch in the pelvic area, chest or throat. Energetic – on swadhisthana or vishuddhi chakra.

Side Leg Stretch (Skandasana)

Level: 1

This final standing posture deepens the stretch to the inside thigh muscles and once again works on balance and awareness.

1. Start in a squatting frog position on the balls of the feet and with the arms hanging straight in front of you, hands just touching the ground.
2. Slide the left foot out to the side as far as comfortable, resting the heel on the ground with the toes and knee pointing straight up.
3. Bring the hands to prayer position in front of the body and lift up through the crown of the head, straightening the spine and putting gentle downward pressure on the pelvis.
4. Remain in this position for up to 30 seconds, breathing normally, extending up through the crown of the head and focusing on balance.
5. When you are ready, place the hands on the ground, step the left foot in and repeat to the other side.

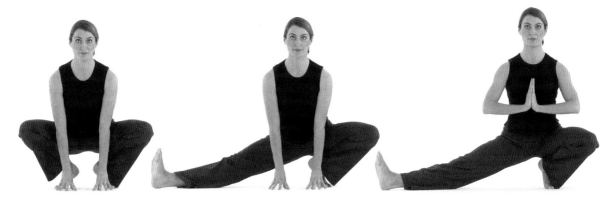

Benefits: This posture stretches and tones the hamstrings and inner thigh muscles. It promotes balance and serenity. The bent knee is strengthened and the spine is stretched. The posture opens the hips.

Common mistakes: The spine should be extended up and not allowed to slouch forward or to either side. The extended leg should be kept straight in alignment with the rotation of your own hip socket. Don't try to force your hip rotation and the leg to the side; it will come in time.

Contraindications: None.

Sequence: During any practice of standing postures.

Awareness: Physical – on balance and a lengthened spine. Energetic – on mooladhara and anahata chakra.

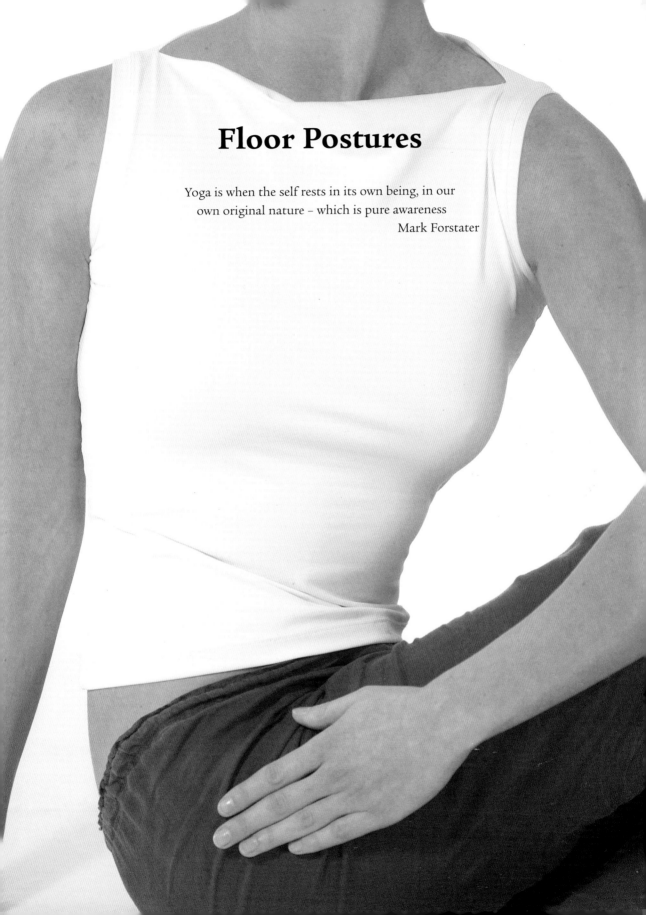

Floor Postures

Yoga is when the self rests in its own being, in our
own original nature – which is pure awareness

Mark Forstater

Postures done from a seated or lying position make up what is also known as the floor sequence. These are usually practised when the body is warmer, stronger and more flexible. The Sun Salutation and standing poses will help your body reach this state. When practising the sitting postures it is vital that you are able to sit comfortably on the ground with an erect spine. It is for this reason that I have included as a preliminary posture the Staff Pose (dandasana), which should give you an idea of how comfortable you are in sitting. In all sitting postures, it is important to remove excess flesh from underneath the sitting bones in order to have a firm base. To do this, simply raise each buttock and lift the buttock flesh up and out of the way to the side. When you return your buttock to the ground you should feel the floor more, and the knobbly bits, the sitting bones, under the buttocks should be more prominent. When doing the lying postures it is important to feel the spine elongated on the floor with the back of the neck lengthened.

Staff Pose (Dandasana)
Level: 1

The Staff Pose is a strangely difficult posture for beginners. It looks so simple and yet is very hard to perfect in terms of comfort and stability. This posture is simply sitting on your buttocks with the legs extended straight out in front of you. And yet, because for so many of us tight hamstrings and inside thigh muscles limit our forward bending, to feel truly comfortable takes time. However, it is worth spending time just sitting and experimenting with this posture, because as your Staff Pose improves, so too will your forward bending.

1. Sit on your buttocks with the legs straight out in front of you. The legs and feet should be together and the feet should be flexed with toes pointing up.
2. Place the palms on the floor to either side of the hips, fingers pointing forward, and press down through the hands. As you press, straighten the spine and lift up through the crown of the head. Try to lift the chest forward and up.

That's it. Sounds simple, doesn't it? And for some of you it will be as simple as it sounds. However, many people feel weight moving back in this position because of tight hamstrings. If you feel any tendency to fall backwards in this position, or are in any discomfort, then this posture is one to spend a bit of time in each day, just feeling how the body reacts. This pose will be the starting position for most of the floor (sitting) postures and so it should be studied. The common mistakes and benefits should be fairly obvious when you try it. Your awareness should be on lifting up out of the waist.

Seated Forward Bend (Paschimottanasana)
Level: 1

The study of seated or lying postures should always begin with the Seated Forward Bend, just as the Standing Forward Bend is the foundation of all standing postures. The deep stretch given to the spine is why this is called paschimottanasana: the back-stretching pose.

Start in Staff Pose (dandasana).

1. Inhale and lift the arms to the side and above the head, palms facing each other. Extend up through the fingers so that you feel the stretch down the side of the body; your upper body is lifting up out of the waist. Press down through the buttocks.
2. Exhale and, leading with the hands, fold forward from the hips. Allow the forward extension of the arms to lead you down into the posture, keeping the spine lengthened.
3. When you have gone forward and down as far as possible, relax the spine and take hold of the legs wherever is comfortable. You may be able to take hold of the feet, touch the toes, or maybe just place the hands on the shins. Whatever is comfortable for you, surrender into the position – don't collapse but relax. Draw backwards through the hips to open and ground the pose.
4. Use the breathing to take you further into the posture. On each inhalation, think of the head moving forward and away from the waist, straightening and extending the spine and lengthening the front of the body. As you do this you should feel the stretch in the hamstrings. With each exhalation relax the body without slouching or bringing curvature to the spine, and find yourself going deeper into the pose.

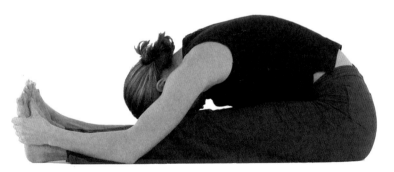

5. Remain in the posture for as long as you are comfortable.
6. When you are ready, inhale and extend forward through the arms and begin lifting them back up. Allow the lift of the arms to guide the rest of the body back to the starting position.

Beginner's variation

For those with extremely tight hamstrings, this forward bend may be challenging. You could use a strap or a pair of very long socks to help you. Place the strap around the soles of the feet with each end resting on the ground near your knees. Go through the steps of the forward bend until you feel that you cannot go any further without slouching the back. At this point take hold of each end of the strap (or sock) and pull against it, using the tension to lengthen the spine and hamstrings. Make sure you keep your arms and elbows in towards the body: this will engage the side body muscles to assist you deeper into the pose. Keep on drawing the chest forwards and the shoulders back. If you continue to use the breathing as explained above and maintain length in the spine you will begin to feel the hamstrings engage and, in time, lengthen.

Benefits: The posture gives an intense stretch to the hamstrings and the entire back and spine. Increases flexibility in the hip joints. Tones and massages the whole pelvic and abdominal area, including the liver, pancreas, spleen, kidneys and adrenal glands. It removes excess fat from that area and helps to alleviate ailments of the uro-genital system. It is good for prolapse and menstrual ailments.

Common mistakes: Slouching into bend instead of elongating the spine as you descend. The knees should remain straight throughout, thighs pressing down. Feet should remain flexed and upright with no twists. Another mistake is poking the chin and face forward – keep the neck relaxed and lengthened at the back. Do not hunch the shoulders but keep them relaxed and moving away from the ears. Do not pull yourself with the hands, instead use the muscles down the side of the body and hips to bend forward gradually, with the hands to guide you as opposed to pull you.

Contraindications: People with slipped disc, sciatica and other diagnosed back problems should avoid this posture.

Sequence: As part of a floor sequence of sitting postures or following inverted work. Should never follow a backward bend due to the extreme nature of the spinal stretch. (To follow a backward bend with a forward bend of this type would put great pressure on the vertebral discs.)

Awareness: Physical – on extension of the spine and folding forward over the legs. Energetic – on swadhisthana chakra.

Butterfly (Baddha Konasana)
Level: 1

The Butterfly is a hip-opening posture. The most important thing about the Butterfly is to be relaxed, and not to force the knees lower than they can go naturally.
Start in Staff Pose (dandasana).

1. Bend the knees and draw them in towards the body so that the soles of the feet are on the floor.
2. Allow the knees to release out to the sides and try to bring the soles of the feet together into a prayer position, with the toes pointing away from the body. The hands should be flat on the ground behind the hips, and pressing down to lengthen the spine.
3. Take hold of the ankles, feet or shins, wherever is comfortable, with each hand. The heels should be a comfortable distance away from the groin; for most people bringing the heels closer intensifies the stretch.
4. Lengthen the spine and press the shoulders down away from the ears. Keep lifting up from the chest. Imagine an invisible string attached to the breastbone and the chest being drawn forwards. Allow the knees to move down towards the ground, touching the ground if possible, and then bring them back up to starting. Imagine a butterfly's wings flapping.
5. Continue this flapping motion with the knees at a steady, rhythmic pace. Keep the spine extended and do not force the knees lower than they want to go.
6. Continue for up to a minute, breathing normally.

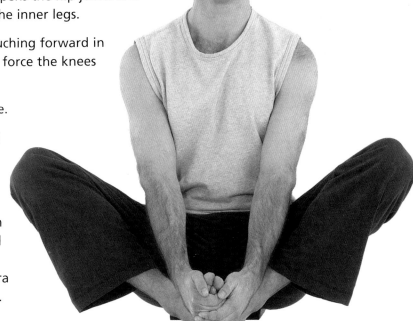

Benefits: The Butterfly opens the hip joints and stretches the muscles of the inner legs.

Common mistakes: Slouching forward in the posture and trying to force the knees down.

Contraindications: None.

Sequence: After forward bending seated postures or before any intense hip openers.

Awareness: Physical – on relaxation of the legs and opening of the hips. Energetic – on mooladhara and swadhisthana chakra.

Single-leg Forward Bend (Janu Sirsasana)
Level: 1

This posture is similar to the Seated Forward Bend but involves tucking one foot in and bending down over one leg only.
Start in Staff Pose (dandasana).

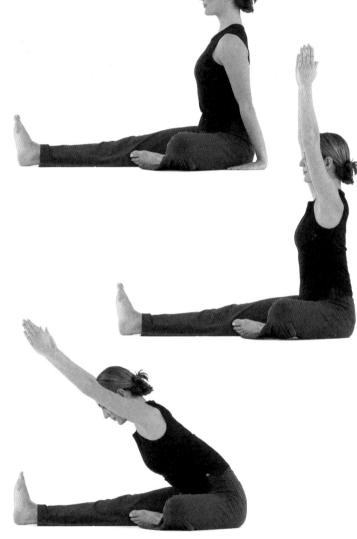

1. Bend the left knee and place the sole of the left foot on the inside of the right thigh. The left knee should be allowed to drop towards the ground.

2. Inhale and lift the arms to the side and above the head, palms facing each other. Extend up through the fingers so that you feel the stretch down the side of the body, as if your upper body is pulling out of the waist. Press down through the buttocks.

3. Exhale and, leading with the hands, fold forward from the hips. Allow the forward extension of the arms to lead you down into the posture, keeping the spine and front body lengthened.

4. When you have gone forward and down as far as possible, relax the spine and take hold wherever is comfortable. You might be able to take hold of the right foot, touch the toes of the right foot or just place the hands on the right shin, or maybe you will need your strap. Do whatever is comfortable for you. Surrender into the position – don't collapse but relax. Also, draw backwards through the hips to open and ground the pose further.

5. Use the breathing to take you further into the posture. On each inhalation, think of the head moving forward and away from the waist, lengthening the front body while straightening and extending the spine. As you do this you should feel the stretch in the hamstrings. With each exhalation relax the body more deeply without slouching or bringing curvature to the spine.

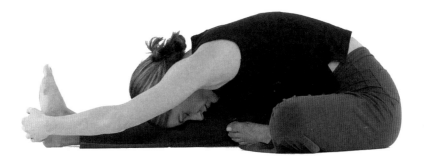

6. Remain in the posture for as long as you are comfortable.
7. When you are ready, inhale and extend forward through the arms and begin lifting them back up. Allow the lift of the arms to guide the rest of the body back to the starting position.
8. Repeat to the other side.

Advanced variation

A variation of this posture is to sit on one heel. This can be quite extreme for some people but generally allows you to move deeper into the stretch. The only difference to the posture as explained above is that from the Staff Pose you should bend the left knee and lift the left buttock off the ground. Then tuck the foot under so that the toes point directly behind you and the heel points up. Sit back on the heel and then continue into the posture. Repeat on both sides.

> **Benefits:** As for Seated Forward Bend, with additional opening of the hip joints as a loosener for sitting poses.

> **Common mistakes:** As for Seated Forward Bend. There is also greater risk of the hips moving out of alignment in this posture due to the one bent leg. Keep the hips square over the extended leg.

> **Contraindications:** As for Seated Forward Bend.

> **Sequence:** As part of a floor or forward bending sequence. Can be practised as preparation for Seated Forward Bend.

> **Awareness:** Physical – as for Seated Forward Bend. Energetic – as for Seated Forward Bend.

Inclined Plane (Purvottanasana)

Level: 1

The Inclined Plane is a traditional counterpose of the forward bending postures in the floor sequence of sitting postures. It gives an intense stretch to the back in the opposite direction to that of the forward bends described on the previous pages.

Start in Staff Pose (dandasana).

1. Move the arms behind you and place the hands flat on the ground about 15cm (6 inches) behind your hips. The fingers should be pointing forward towards the buttocks.

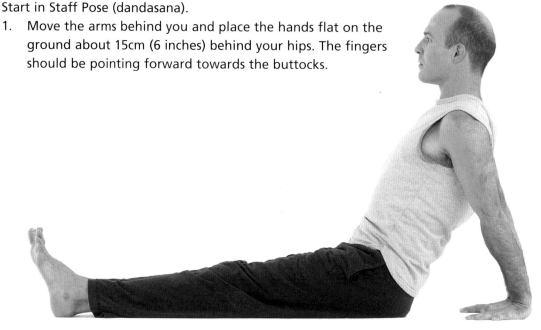

2. Pressing the palms into the ground and pointing the toes down so that the soles of the feet move towards the ground, inhale, and keeping the legs straight lift the hips up into the air. Stretch the neck and release the head back as far as comfortable.

3. Breathing normally, try to take the toes to the ground and continue to lift the hips, abdomen and chest to the sky.

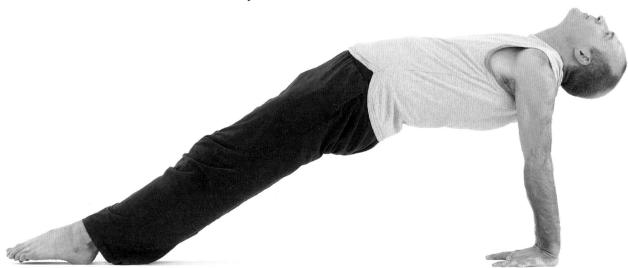

4. Hold for up to 10 deep breaths and then relax the buttocks back down to the ground.
5. Relax in the Staff Pose.

Beginner's variation

This posture can also be done with bent knees from the Staff Pose if the basic inclined plane is too extreme. In this variation the hands should remain down alongside the body, palms pressing into the ground by the hips. Once again lift the hips, but this time press away with the knees so that the soles of the feet come to the ground but the knees remain bent.

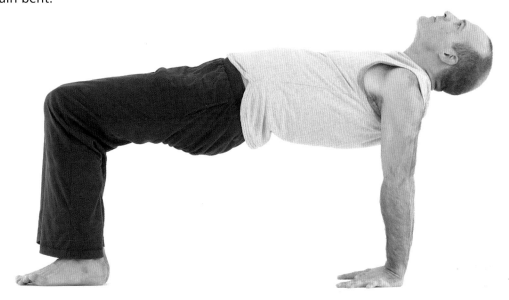

Benefits: Strengthens the shoulders, arms and wrists. Gives a deep stretch to the front of the body from the neck to the toes. Tones the lumbar/lower area of the spine, the buttocks, the legs and the Achilles tendon. Opens the chest to encourage deep breathing. Rejuvenates and loosens the neck.

Common mistakes: In the full Inclined Plane, bending the knees. This should only be done intentionally in the beginner's variation. Not engaging the shoulders, hollowing the chest. The upper body should be pulling up as much as possible. Bending the elbows and straining the neck. Not pressing the toes towards the ground.

Contraindications: Those with high blood pressure, heart problems and stomach ulcers should avoid this posture.

Sequence: Following forward bending postures or during backbending sequence.

Awareness: Physical – on the lift and length of the body. Energetic – on manipura chakra.

Cradling Lotus

Level: 1

I use Cradling Lotus as preparation for sitting postures that are used in meditation (see pages 166-7). However, it is also wonderful as an opener before continuing to the more intense postures in the floor sequence (sitting postures). That is why the posture is here, although you should feel free to use it independently before any long period of sitting. Start in Staff Pose (dandasana).

1. Bend the right leg and draw the knee into the chest, sole of the foot on the floor. Your right hand should be holding the front of the right knee, palm facing in.
2. Release the knee out to the side as if you are doing a half Butterfly, keeping the right hand in place. Take the left hand underneath the outside of the right foot.
2. Lift the right foot off the floor, lengthen the spine and then gently rock the knee in a side-to-side motion. Visualize rocking a baby in your arms. Maintain pressure down through the left thigh throughout, foot flexed.
4. Continue 'rocking the baby' for up to a minute, breathing normally.
5. When ready, release the right leg and repeat to other side.

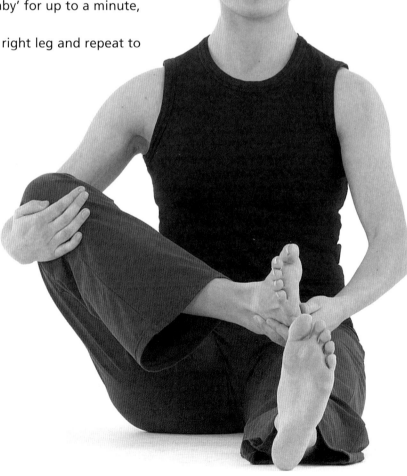

90

Advanced Variation I

From the step 2 above, release the right arm and wrap it around the right leg so that the knee of the right leg is pressing into the inside of the right elbow. Release the left arm and wrap it around the right foot so that the foot is resting on the inside of the left elbow joint. Try to interlock or hold the hands together. If you cannot do this, simply bring the hands as close as possible together, palms pressing into the outside of the right leg. Start 'rocking the baby'.

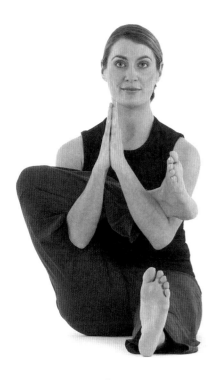

Advanced Variation II

From the step 2 above, take the right hand and thread it through the inside of the right leg so that the leg is hooked on the right elbow crease. Release the left hand and take it under the right foot so that the foot rests on the left elbow crease. Bring the palms together in a prayer position if you can. Start 'rocking the baby'.

Benefits: The posture is a great hip opener and the variations also give the backs of the thighs and buttocks an additional stretch.

Common mistakes: Slouching forward in the posture and forcing the leg to 'rock' more than is comfortable.

Contraindications: None.

Sequence: As part of a seated sequence, especially as preparation for the more advanced hip-opening exercises. As a preparation for sitting postures.

Awareness: Physical – on relaxing the legs and lengthening the spine. On moving in a steady rhythm. Energetic – on mooladhara and swadhisthana chakra.

Seated Wide Leg Bend (Upavista Konasana)

Level: 2

The Seated Wide Leg Bend is the posture that causes the most grimaces among beginning yoga students. A huge amount of flexibility in the hips and groin area is required to master it and many students have trouble even opening their legs beyond a 90-degree angle. Just open the legs as much as comfortable and keep gently working at it.
Start in Staff Pose (dandasana).

1. Open the legs out to each side as far as comfortable. The feet are flexed. Place the hands flat on the ground directly behind you and push through the palms, lengthening the spine. Try to become comfortable in this position.
2. Inhale and lift the arms to the sides then above the head, palms facing each other. Lift up through the fingers so you can feel the stretch down the sides of the body. Lengthen the spine.

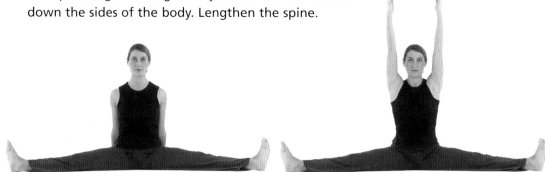

3. Exhale and fold forward from the waist, leading with the hands. Go as far as is comfortable. (If you are not comfortable leading with the arms then just walk the hands forward on the floor, little by little, keeping your spine as straight as possible.) If you have very little flexibility in this posture then go as far as possible before placing the hands on the ground in front of you to balance yourself. Use the breathing to keep extending forward and attempt gradually to move deeper into the posture.
4. If you can, keep folding until your forehead eventually reaches the ground in front of you, stretching the arms along the ground ahead, palms down, curling the tailbone under to ensure that your buttocks stay on the ground.

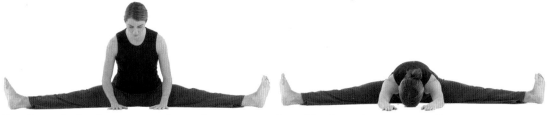

5. Remain in the posture for as long as comfortable, breathing normally.
6. When you are ready, walk your hands back until your torso is once again in an upright position.
7. Exhale and bend the body to the right, keeping your body square to the front. Bring the right arm down and try to take hold of the foot, or the leg where comfortable,

if possible with the elbow on the ground. Keep the left arm in line with the ears and stretch through the fingers, extending the arm and stretching one side of the body. Try to take the left arm down so it is parallel to the ground. If you cannot reach the foot you can always place a strap around it and hold on to both ends of the strap with your lower hand.

8. Remain in the posture for up to 30 seconds, breathing normally. Inhale and bring the left hand back to vertical and straighten the torso. Repeat to the other side.

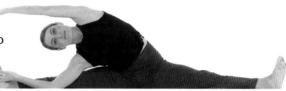

Beginner's variation: Single Seated Wide Leg Bend (Parivrtta Janu Sirsasana)
In this variation the movements are the same as above except that they are done with one leg tucked into the groin, and one leg extended as wide as comfortable. Begin by opening both legs as far as comfortable. Then bend the left leg at the knee, tucking the heel into the groin. The left knee should be allowed to drop to the ground. Straighten yourself up as much as possible. From this point repeat the movements described in the Seated Wide Leg Bend. After finishing, change the legs over and repeat to the other side.

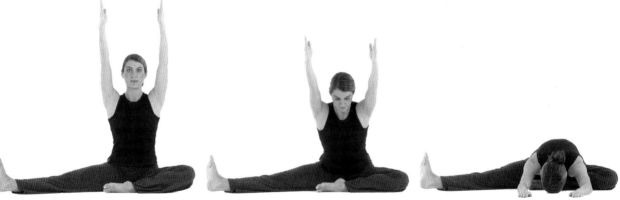

Benefits: As for the Seated Forward Bend with an additional deep stretch for the inner thighs and hip joints and toning for the side body.

Common mistakes: Legs rolling in – keep the legs flat on the ground with the kneecaps and toes pointing up. Do not take the legs too wide; go as far as you are comfortable. Other common mistakes are similar to Seated Forward Bend.

Contraindications: As with Seated Forward Bend.

Sequence: As part of a forward bending or seated sequence.

Awareness: Physical – on opening the hips and lengthening the upper body. Energetic – on mooladhara or swadhisthana chakra.

Double Pigeon (Dwi Pada Rajakapotasana)

Level: 3

This is an intense stretch that should never be done without a sufficient warm-up. Start in Staff Pose (dandasana).

1. Bend the left leg and place it under the right leg so that the upper part of the left ankle is directly under the right knee; the foot should protrude from the side. If you look down, a triangle should be formed between the legs.

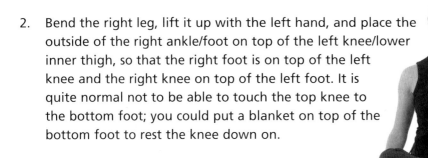

2. Bend the right leg, lift it up with the left hand, and place the outside of the right ankle/foot on top of the left knee/lower inner thigh, so that the right foot is on top of the left knee and the right knee on top of the left foot. It is quite normal not to be able to touch the top knee to the bottom foot; you could put a blanket on top of the bottom foot to rest the knee down on.

3. Press the hands down behind your hips to lengthen the spine. On an inhalation take the arms up straight above you, palms facing each other.

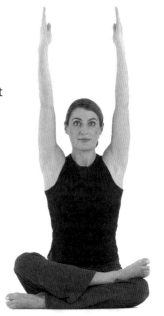

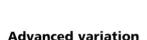

4. On an exhalation lower the arms in front of the body and place the elbows on top of the right foot and right knee, pressing down and bringing the hands together in prayer position. This can be a real pleasure/pain position for many, so breathe deeply, relax the body and release the hips. Hold the position for as long as comfortable, breathing normally.

Advanced variation

To go further into the position – but only if the above is comfortable – bring the hands to the floor in front of you and walk them forward. Slowly bend from the hips and continue to move forward until the forearms are on the floor. Breathe deeply and relax. If possible, release the head towards the floor, walking the hands further forward, straightening the arms if possible and taking the forehead all the way to the ground. Keep the spine lengthened and feel the buttocks on the ground throughout. To come out of this pose retrace your steps until the spine is erect again.

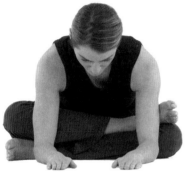
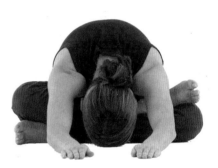

5. To come out of the posture, lift the top leg out of the pose, straighten the pose and give the legs a really good and vigorous shake.
6. Repeat to the other side.

Benefits: This posture gives a delightful/intense/deep (depending on your level) stretch to the hips, thighs, knees and ankles. Combined with the forward bend it stretches the spine and prepares the body for sitting in Full Lotus position.

Common mistakes: Improper alignment of the legs to begin with. If you are unable to go into the full posture to begin with, it is better only to go as far as you can and then simply relax the body rather than to force the knees down or do anything that might cause intense pain.

Contraindications: Those with knee problems should approach with great caution.

Sequence: Following Seated Wide Leg Bends or as preparation for sitting postures.

Awareness: Physical – on relaxing the legs and buttocks and opening the hips. Energetic – on mooladhara and swadhisthana chakra.

Cow's Face Posture (Gomukhasana)
Level: 3

As with the Double Pigeon, this is another great stretch of the thighs and hips. Do not force yourself into this posture and make sure you are warm before attempting it. Start in Staff Pose (dandasana).

1. Bend the left leg back and across so the knee is directly in front of you and on the ground. The heel should be tucked under the right buttock, toes pointing out. Press the hands down into the ground behind your hips to straighten the spine.

2. Bend the right knee and bring the foot to the ground on the outside of the left knee. Hold the right foot and guide the right foot back so that the right knee begins to come down towards the left knee. Eventually you want the knees to be on top of each other, outside edges of the feet on the ground with the spine erect.

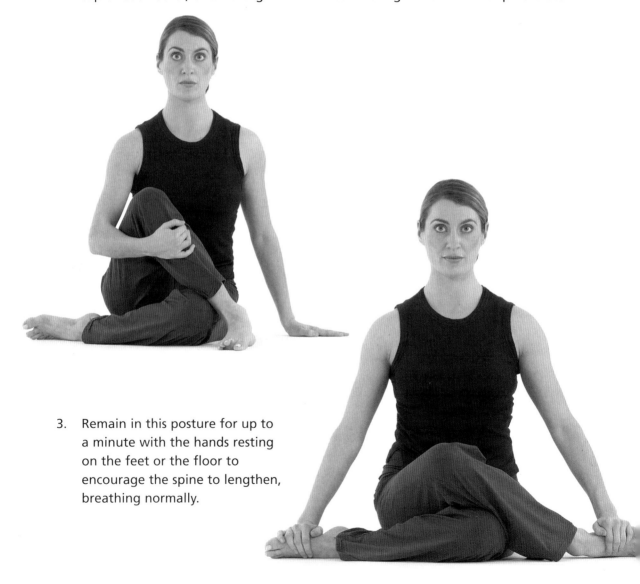

3. Remain in this posture for up to a minute with the hands resting on the feet or the floor to encourage the spine to lengthen, breathing normally.

Advanced variation

When you are comfortable in the basic posture, then you can intensify the stretch, bringing the back, shoulders and arms into the pose. Sitting comfortably in the Cow's Face, lift the right arm to the sky and bend the elbow so that you reach as far down your back with the hand as possible. Bend the left arm, take the hand behind the back and try to take hold of the right hand. If the hands are joined, lift the right elbow upwards to stretch both arms and shoulders and continue to lengthen the spine. Sit comfortably for up to a minute, breathing normally. If you are unable to link the hands, then practise this arm movement in a normal sitting posture using a strap or sock, holding it in the right hand so that it dangles down your back. Take hold of the strap wherever you can with the left hand and pull up with the right elbow, stretching the left shoulder and shortening the distance between the hands. When you are eventually able to take hold of the hands then try the movement again in Cow's Face.

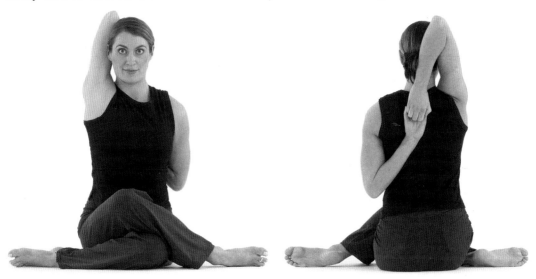

4. To release from the posture simply unfold the legs and relax the body in Staff Pose (dandasana).
5. Repeat to the other side.

Benefits: This posture gives a delightful/intense/deep (depending on your level) stretch to the hips, thighs, knees and ankles. It cures cramp in the legs and makes them feel elongated.

Common mistakes: As with Double Pigeon.

Contraindications: Those with knee problems should approach with great caution.

Sequence: Following Seated Wide Leg Bends or as preparation for sitting postures.

Awareness: Physical – on relaxing the legs and extending the spine. Energetic – on mooladhara and swadhisthana chakra.

Half Spinal Twist (Ardha Matsyendrasana)
Level: 1–2

The Half Spinal Twist is one of the few postures in this book that deal with the twisting of the spinal column as a main feature. There are some more twisting postures in the backward bending sequence.

Begin by sitting on your heels with your hands resting on your thighs.

1. Shift your buttocks to the left side of the heels and sit down on the ground.

2. Take the right leg over the left thigh and place the right foot on the ground so that it touches the left side of the left thigh, near the knee. Try to place both buttocks on the ground. Place the right hand flat down on the ground directly behind the tailbone, fingers pointing away from you. Inhale and raise the left arm into the air, fingers pointing up.

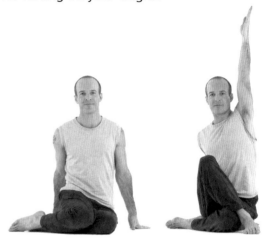

3. Exhale and bring the left arm across the body so that it moves to the right-hand side of the right thigh. Try to wedge the left elbow against the right thigh. If possible wedge it to such an extent that you can straighten the left arm and reach down and take hold of the right ankle. As you press your left elbow into the right thigh, rotate the torso to the right so that your shoulders open to the side and you begin to look behind you. If you are unable to straighten the arm and hold the ankle then simply press the left elbow into the right thigh and hold your left hand straight up, fingers pointing towards the sky.

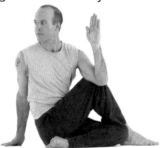 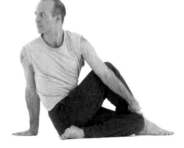

4. With each inhalation try to straighten the spine so that you are not leaning back at all. Lift up through the crown of the head and lengthen the neck. With each exhalation try to rotate the torso just a little bit more.

5. Hold the posture for up to a minute, breathing deeply.

6. When you are ready to come out of the posture, release the left elbow from the right thigh and inhale the left arm straight up. Rotate the body back to centre. Sit back onto your heels for a few moments before repeating on the opposite side.

Beginner's variation

Instead of beginning by sitting on the heels, begin in Staff Pose, dandasana. Bend the right knee and bring the foot across so that it is placed on the ground on the left-hand side of the left knee. Take the right hand and place it behind the tailbone, approximately 15–20cm (6–8 inches) away from the buttocks. Inhale and lift the left arm straight up. Bring the left arm across and wedge the elbow against the right-hand side of thigh, just across and below the knee. Pressing the left elbow against the right thigh, rotate the body to the right so that you look behind you. Hold for up to 30 seconds then release the left elbow, inhale as the arm rises straight up and rotate back to centre. Repeat on the other side.

Advanced variation

Go through the steps of the Half Spinal Twist until you are fully rotated. Lift the hand from the floor behind you and take it behind the back as much as possible. Release the grip on the ankle and take your other arm through the leg, trying to take hold of the hand behind the body. Lift up and straighten the body. Hold for up to 30 seconds. Repeat on the other side.

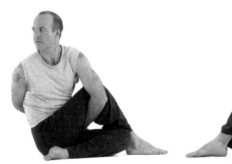

Benefits: This posture stretches the muscles on one side of the back and abdomen while contracting the muscles on the other side. It tones the nerves of the spine and makes the back supple. It is beneficial for cases of slipped disc. It massages the abdominal organs, alleviating digestive ailments.

Common mistakes: The upper body should not fall backwards – keep lengthening up through the spine. The buttocks should move towards the ground, even if this is not possible to achieve at first. The breathing should never stop, but should be used to deepen the rotation of the spine.

Contraindications: Pregnant women or people with a diagnosed back condition should not practise this posture.

Sequence: This posture may be practised after forward bending or backbending postures or as part of a floor sequence of sitting postures.

Awareness: Physical – on the twist and stretch of the body. Energetic – on manipura chakra.

Downward Dog (Adho Mukha Svanasana)
Level: 1–2

The Downward Dog (also called the Inverted V, which is the shape you should picture the body making in the posture) is a difficult pose to classify. Because the head is below the heart many people would class it as an inverted posture, but for the sake of this book I have chosen to place it in the floor sequence of sitting postures. Either way it is an important and dynamic posture to learn.

Begin on your hands and knees, with the wrists directly below the shoulders and the knees below the hips. The toes should be turned under so that heels are pointing up.

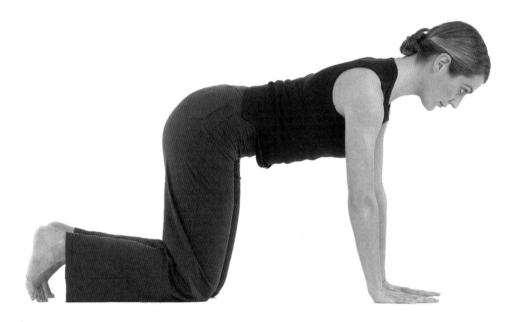

1. Press down through the palms of the hands, spreading the fingers out on the ground.
2. Inhale, then exhale and lift the hips up, straighten the legs and press down through the backs of the legs and the heels. (Don't worry if your heels aren't on the ground. This will come with practice.) Press down through the palms, keeping the arms straight. Lengthen through the back of the neck as you draw the chin down slightly. Keep the neck relaxed.
3. Keep the legs and the feet parallel. Try to press the heels to the ground and extend through the balls of the feet. Press your shins back and release your calves. Firm the thighs to stretch evenly through the hamstrings and try to lengthen the tailbone as you lift the lower belly. Keep your lower ribs soft also.
4. Any adjustments needed to the posture should be done by moving the feet; the hands should remain exactly where they began, pressing the ground away.

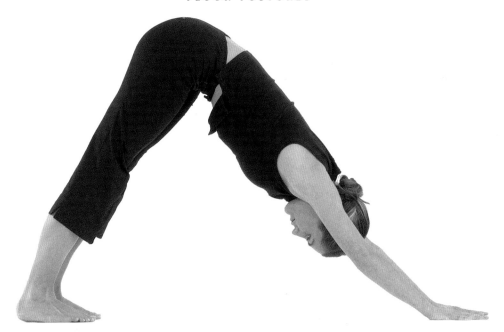

5. Keep lifting the hips. Imagine balloons attached to the buttocks lifting them up into the air. Lift the abdomen and soften the shoulders, opening the chest.
6. Hold the position for up to 30 seconds, breathing normally.
7. To come out of the posture simply lower the knees to the ground. Relax the buttocks down to the heels and stretch the arms forward, relaxing your forehead to the ground or go into Child's Pose. Repeat up to five times.

Benefits: This posture, surprisingly, removes fatigue and restores lost energy. It gives a deep stretch to the hamstrings and tones the legs. It loosens the ankles. The shoulders are opened and arms and wrists strengthened. The spine is stretched and toned. As the diaphragm is lifted, the heartbeat is slowed, massaging the internal organs and revitalizing the body.

Common mistakes: The knees should not be bent in the full position. Weight should not be forward over the hands but rather moving back and up towards the hips, then down and back through the heels. The arms should be firm but the elbows should not lock. The hips and buttocks should not sag downward. Release any tension in the neck.

Contraindications: None.

Sequence: This is one of the most versatile of all postures. It can be used as part of a floor sequence (sitting postures), at the beginning or end of a practice or as a posture to link all other postures.

Awareness: Physical – on lifting the hips, opening the chest and taking the weight back and up; on sinking the heels to the ground. Energetic – on vishuddhi chakra.

Crow (Bakasana)

Level: 2

The Crow is a balancing posture that requires a fair amount of care and upper body strength, though nowhere near as much as most people seem to think when they see someone in the full posture. The Crow is all about slowly finding the point of balance where the feet simply lift from the ground and all of the weight is gracefully taken by the arms and wrists. If you are concerned about this posture, try putting a couple of pillows in front of you so that if you fall, your head will fall onto something soft. For many people, when the fear of harming themselves goes, the posture suddenly becomes that much easier.

1. Start squatting down on the balls of the feet with your hands flat on the ground in front of you. The hands should be in line and a little wider than shoulder-width. The fingers may be pointing in slightly or pointing straight ahead, spread.

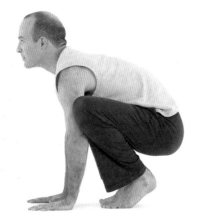 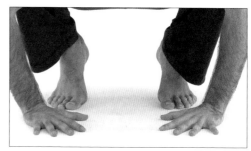

2. Bend the elbows so that the upper part of the arm forms a platform for the legs to rest on. Tighten the abdominal muscles and move towards the tips of your toes and place the shins on the upper arms with the knees facing out. Adjust the shins so that they feel comfortable on the upper arms. Find a point of focus on the ground in front of you.

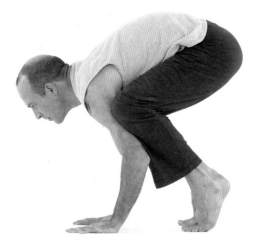 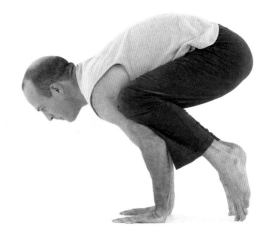

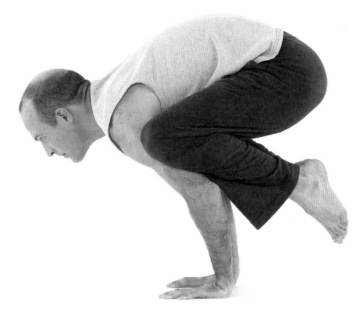

3. Exhale, lift the hips up, move the body forward slowly, transferring weight onto your hands and feel the toes beginning to lift from the ground until eventually only the big toes touch. If you feel yourself falling forward, take the weight back again onto the toes. Try moving forward again, keeping the head up and attempting to find the point where the toes lift off the ground and the body is balanced, with all the weight being supported through the wrists and hands.
4. Try to push down through the arms and hands, straightening them slightly and lifting the body higher. Visualize a string lifting the middle of the back.
5. Hold for about 30 seconds or up to a minute, breathing normally.
6. When you are ready to come out of the posture simply allow your weight to move back and let your toes come back to the ground.

Benefits: This posture strengthens the wrists, arms and shoulders. Confidence is increased through the ability to balance. The abdominal muscles are also strengthened through contraction. Concentration is improved.

Common mistakes: Proper balancing is essential to this posture and too many beginners try to move forward or hop into the crow too quickly, resulting in loss of balance. Remember this a gradual transfer of weight from back to front. The shins should be high up on the arms, and firmly placed so that they do not slip off. Dropping the head is also a mistake: keep a point of focus ahead.

Contraindications: Those with any history of wrist problems or dislocated shoulders should not attempt this posture.

Sequence: Varied but can be integrated with standing postures after the body is warm.

Awareness: Physical – on balance, breathing and the strength of the arms. Energetic – on anahata chakra.

Side Angle Crow (Parsva Bakasana)
Level: 2

This posture is similar to the Crow but in this variation both legs balance on one arm and the weight is not evenly distributed. However, if you are able to do the Crow then in time you will also be able to do this posture.

1. Start squatting down on the balls of the feet with your hands flat on the ground in front of you. The hands should be in line and a little wider than shoulder-width. The fingers may be pointing in slightly or pointing straight ahead, spread.

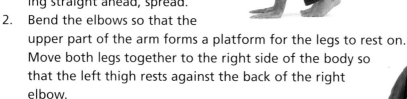

2. Bend the elbows so that the upper part of the arm forms a platform for the legs to rest on. Move both legs together to the right side of the body so that the left thigh rests against the back of the right elbow.

3. Lift the legs up onto the back of the right upper arm so that the left thigh is resting on the arm and the right leg is on top of the left leg. Engage the abdominal muscles.

4. Exhale, lift the hips up, move the body forward slowly and feel the toes beginning to lift from the ground. If you feel yourself falling forward, take the weight back again onto the toes. Try moving forward again, keeping the head up and attempting to find the point where the toes lift off the ground and the body is balanced, with all the weight being supported through the wrists. This will be more extreme through one arm than the other because of the downward pressure of the legs.

5. Try to push down through the arms, straightening them slightly and lifting the body higher.

6. Hold for about 30 seconds or up to a minute, breathing normally.

7. When you are ready to come out of the posture, simply allow your weight to move back and let your toes come back to the ground.

Benefits: As for Crow on previous page.

Common mistakes: As for Crow.

Contraindications: As for Crow.

Sequence: Practise after the Crow.

Awareness: As for Crow.

Backward Bending Postures

Moments of life are gift-wrapped in bright colours.

Anon

Backward bending postures turn the body out to face the world. They generally expand the chest, opening the heart, and encourage inhalation, and therefore are associated with life and the embrace of happiness. These postures are primarily stimulating and prepare you for activity and motion. They stretch and tone the abdominal muscles and create flexibility and improved circulation for the spine and surrounding muscles, alleviating back problems and bringing health and vitality to our movements.

For these postures, proper alignment and form are vital. This is because of the potential stress to the lower back that can be caused by improper practice. Take your time learning these postures and make sure to read and re-read the instructions for each one in turn before and after you practise. An important note is always to focus on extension of the spine in all the postures shown in this section. This may seem strange to say, given that most of the postures involve some form of backbend. However, the extension I am talking about here is a subtle extension in which the different parts of the body move away from each other, forward or backwards, during the stretch, creating space in which the back and spine can arch. Never simply lift into one of these postures without first picturing the way the different parts of the body are pulling away from each other. Study the pictures in detail to observe this point.

Backward bending postures are among the most rewarding and beautiful postures in yoga, but also among the most demanding. I am certain, however, that once you become more comfortable in each of the backbending postures, you will begin to see the huge benefits they can bring to your everyday life.

Cobra (Bhujangasana)
Level: 1

The Cobra rears up its head to defend against predators, so too will this posture help to fight against a variety of ailments. In many ways it is the most important of all backbending postures, since it prepares the spine for all the following movements in this section.

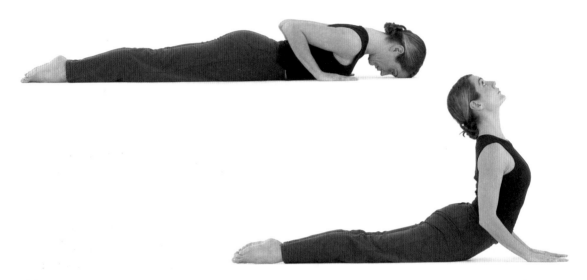

1. Begin by lying flat on your abdomen with the legs straight and feet together, soles of the feet facing up. Make a pillow by placing one hand on top of the other, palms down and elbows out, and rest your head on the pillow, looking in either direction. Relax and take a few deep breaths.
2. Place the palms of the hands flat on the floor underneath the shoulders (fingers pointing forward so that the tips of the fingers are approximately in line with the front of the shoulders), with the elbows pointing back and tucked into the side of the body.
3. Rest the forehead on the ground and relax the body.
4. Inhale and slowly begin to lift the head, neck and shoulders forward and up off the ground, moving the heart forward and engaging the back muscles to bend upward. Continue to lift up as far as is comfortable without putting any weight down through the hands. Keep the weight pressing down through the pelvic area and the legs extended backwards and feet together, flat on the ground.
5. When you have lifted as high as is comfortable using only the back muscles, begin to press down through the palms and engage the arm muscles to lift you further up. Keep the elbows partially bent and tucked into the side of the body (never lock the elbows and straighten the arms completely in the Cobra) and press the shoulders down and back, away from the ears, avoiding any hunching of the shoulders. Tilt the head slightly back so that the chin points upward. The pubic bone should be in contact with the ground throughout.

6. Breathe comfortably in the final posture and continually try to press the shoulders down and back away from the ears, opening the chest and lifting the heart towards the sky.

Advanced variation – King Cobra

From the normal Cobra, part the knees slightly and bend the knees and bring the toes together. Walk the hands back and straighten the arms, making sure your shoulders stay down. Begin arching back and feel the pubic area lifting off the floor. Release the head backwards, trying to touch the tips of the toes behind you.

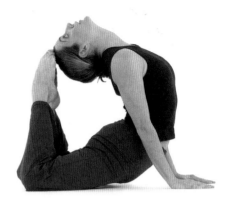

7. To come out of the posture, exhale and slowly bend the arms and lower the torso to the ground, extending forward as you come down with the chin, nose and forehead brushing to the ground to finish.

The Cobra can be an extreme posture for beginners. It is best to attempt the posture in short bursts rather than tire yourself trying to hold the posture for too long, especially as fatigue can produce poor alignment of the body. Think of the upper body reaching forward and up towards the sky, and the lower back curving gracefully from the tailbone to the neck.

Benefits: The Cobra can relocate slipped discs, remove backache and keep the spine supple and healthy. It tones the ovaries, and alleviates menstrual and other gynaecological ailments. The Cobra stimulates the appetite, alleviates constipation and is hugely beneficial as a massage for the internal organs. The arms, back and shoulders are strengthened.

Common mistakes: Too often students lift straight up without any extended forward movement of the upper body: this risks compression of the spine. Feet should not be allowed to drift apart and the legs should be kept firmly on the ground with a feeling of extension backwards. Always maintain a subtle bend at the elbows even at the highest point.

Contraindications: Those with peptic ulcers, hernia or hyperthyroidism should avoid the Cobra.

Sequence: As the beginning of a backbending sequence, at the peak of your practise allowing the previous postures to warm and prepare the spine.

Awareness: Physical – coordinating breathing with movement and developing a smooth arching movement while entering and exiting Cobra. Energetic – on swadhisthana chakra.

Locust (Shalabhjasana)

Level: 2–3

The Full Locust is an extremely demanding posture that requires a lot of flexibility in the spine. Most students would do fine practising only the Intermediate Locust until the point when the legs naturally lift high enough to proceed further. A firm foundation, provided by the arms, is essential. Begin by lying flat on your abdomen with the legs straight and feet together, soles of the feet facing up. Make a pillow by placing one hand on top of the other, palms down and elbows out, and rest your head on the pillow, looking in either direction. Relax and take a few deep breaths.

Preparation for Locust

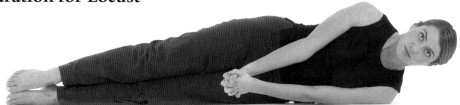

1. Roll onto one side and bring the hands together in front of the groin, as low down on the thighs as possible. The hands may be clenched together or side by side with the palms facing down (beginners usually find that clenching the hands together is easiest).

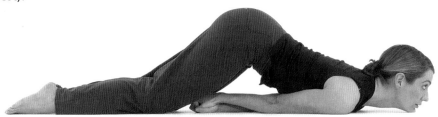

2. Roll back over onto your front and lift the tailbone slightly so that you can work the hands further underneath the body. Rest the chin flat on the ground. The shoulders should be pressed down and back, away from the ears.

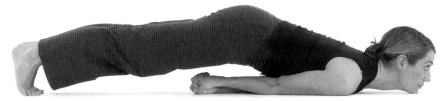

3. Tuck the toes under so that you are on the balls of the feet, with the knees and pelvic area lifted from the ground with straight legs. Push through the arms and the heels to firm your base body.

4. Inhale and lift the right leg as high as possible, trying to keep the leg straight by pushing back through the thighs. Continue to firm your base.
5. Exhale and lower the right leg. Repeat to the other side.
6. Repeat on both sides slowly 3–5 times.

various hand positions for locust

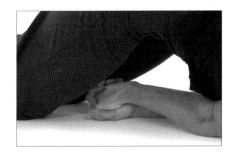

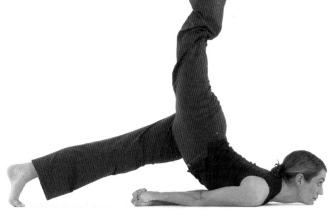

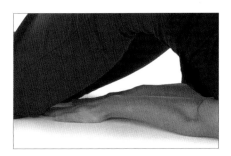

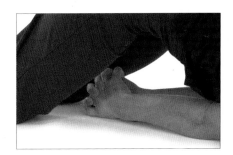

Intermediate Locust

1. With the hands clenched under the body and legs flat on the ground, extend the chin slightly forward on the ground. Close the eyes and relax the body.
2. Inhale and slowly raise both legs together as high as possible, pushing down through the pelvic area and arms and extending forward through the chin. The legs should be kept straight throughout. Higher elevation of the legs is produced by applying further pressure through the arms and contracting the lower back muscles.
3. Hold the posture as long as is comfortable without strain. Breathe normally.
4. Exhale and slowly lower the legs to the ground. Relax the body. Make a pillow with the hands and place the head on the pillow, looking in the opposite direction to the one you started with.

Full Locust

Level: 3

1. Find the same starting position as for the Intermediate Locust.
2. Take three deep breaths, focusing on bringing energy into the body while inhaling and relaxing the body while exhaling.
3. Inhale and press down through the arms while simultaneously tensing the thigh muscles and lifting the legs up from the ground. Arch the back and continue to lift the legs until the pelvic area also lifts off the ground.

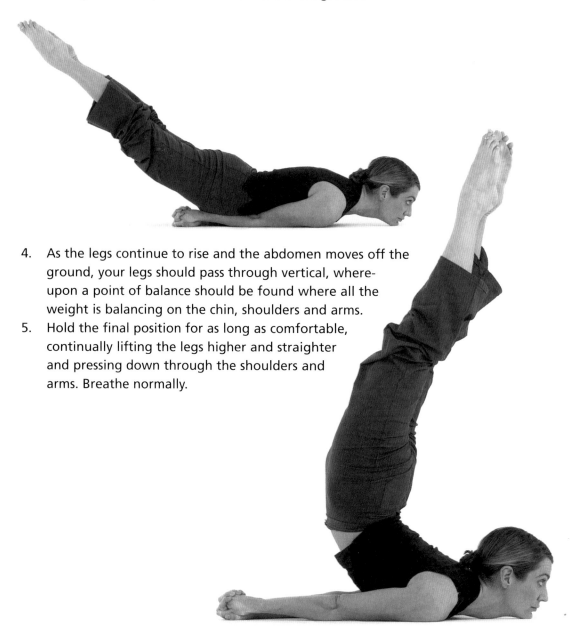

4. As the legs continue to rise and the abdomen moves off the ground, your legs should pass through vertical, whereupon a point of balance should be found where all the weight is balancing on the chin, shoulders and arms.
5. Hold the final position for as long as comfortable, continually lifting the legs higher and straighter and pressing down through the shoulders and arms. Breathe normally.

6. To return to the starting position, slowly lower the legs while retaining the breath, trying to lower each part of the body in turn, i.e. abdomen, pelvis, legs.
7. Make a pillow with the hands and place the head on the pillow, looking in the opposite direction to the one you started with.

The Full Locust is traditionally achieved only when the knees actually bend beyond vertical and the soles of the feet rest on the top of the head. Picture that! For this book, we give that one a miss.

Benefits: The Locust stimulates the entire autonomic nervous system. It strengthens the lower back and tones the sciatic nerves, providing relief from backache, sciatica and slipped disc. Locust tones and balances the functioning of the liver and other abdominal organs. Arms, back and shoulders are strengthened. Buttocks are toned through constant clenching.

Common mistakes: The legs should be kept together and not allowed to drift apart or bend. Far more important than lifting the legs high is keeping the extension down through the legs. The weight should be taken by the arms in the most part, so that the lifting is not done entirely by the lower back, placing extreme pressure on the lower spine. Never allow someone else to lift your legs higher just so you can see how much you can bend – this is potentially dangerous. Allow your own body to dictate how high the legs lift; in time you will find it easier.

Contraindications: Those with heart conditions, high blood pressure or hernia should not practise this posture.

Sequence: During backbending; most beneficial after Cobra and before Bow. At the peak of your practise allowing the previous postures to warm and prepare the spine.

Awareness: Physical – the abdomen, and relaxing the back completely. Energetic – on vishuddhi chakra.

Bow (Dhanurasana)
Level: 1–2

A graceful and deep stretch, the Bow is true to its name. In the bow breathing is vital, and in time it will become so comfortable that you may find yourself rocking back and forward with your breathing while indulging in this remarkable posture.

Beginner's Variation: Preparation for Bow

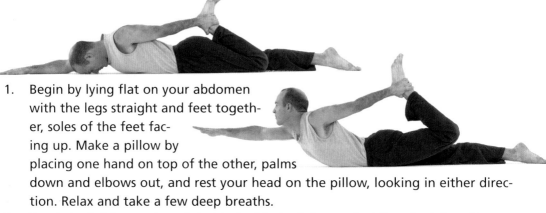

1. Begin by lying flat on your abdomen with the legs straight and feet together, soles of the feet facing up. Make a pillow by placing one hand on top of the other, palms down and elbows out, and rest your head on the pillow, looking in either direction. Relax and take a few deep breaths.
2. Bend the left leg and reach behind with the left arm, holding the left ankle, not the arch of the foot, with the left hand, palm facing in. Extend the right arm flat along the ground in front of you, palm down and fingers pointing away from the head. Rest the forehead on the ground and relax and breathe normally.
3. Inhale and lift the right arm up as high as you can take it, extending forward through the fingers, and engage the lower back muscles so that the head, shoulders and chest also lift off the ground. At the same time, lift your left foot up and away from you and lift the left thigh off the ground. It may be challenging to maintain balance at first: take your time and move into the posture slowly. Remain in the pose, breathing normally, as long as comfortable.
4. When you are ready, lower the left leg to the ground and lower the chest, head and right arm. Release the hold on the left ankle and relax for a few moments. Then repeat on the other side, lifting the left arm and right leg.

Bow

1. Bend both knees and bring the heels close to the buttocks. Reach behind with both arms and hold the ankles, palms facing each other. Drop your shoulders down and back, away from the ears, and straighten the arms. The arms should remain straight throughout the posture; they act

as the string of the bow. Rest the forehead on the ground and relax.

2. Inhale and lift your feet up and away from the body while simultaneously lifting the thighs from the ground. Allow the movement of the feet away from you to act as a lever, pulling your upper body up off the ground. Engage the muscles in your lower back and buttocks and continue the upward movement of the head, shoulders and chest off the ground.

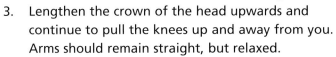
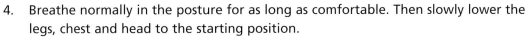

3. Lengthen the crown of the head upwards and continue to pull the knees up and away from you. Arms should remain straight, but relaxed.

4. Breathe normally in the posture for as long as comfortable. Then slowly lower the legs, chest and head to the starting position.

The Bow can be held for as long as possible. However, the exit from the posture should be graceful and controlled. Do not get so fatigued that you allow the legs and upper body to collapse down to the ground; instead, guide the body back to a lying, flat position.

Benefits: The liver and abdominal organs and muscles are massaged and the pancreas and adrenal glands are toned. The kidney is massaged and excess fat around the abdominal area is reduced. The Bow assists digestion, eliminative and reproductive organs, and improves blood circulation. The spinal column is realigned and chest ailments may be reduced. The chest is opened and the shoulders and buttocks are toned, assisting posture. Period pains could be helped for women. Flexibility and strength are encouraged in the spine.

Common mistakes: The body should not be tensed too much as this may compress the spine. Arms should not be bent, but remain straight throughout. Beginners often find it strange to push the feet away from the body throughout, but it is this action that allows us to lift the thighs from the ground. Do not allow the chest to sag, but keep it lifting up and out. It is easier for a beginner to keep the knees apart, but the eventual goal is to have the knees together.

Contraindications: If you have a weak heart, high blood pressure or hernia you should not attempt this posture. The Bow should not be practised before sleeping as it stimulates the adrenal organs.

Sequence: During a backbending sequence. At the peak of your practise allowing the previous postures to warm and prepare the spine.

Awareness: Physical – abdominal area, back or breathing. Energetic – vishuddhi, anahata or manipura chakra.

Camel (Ustrasana)
Level: 2

The Camel can be a very challenging posture for beginners simply because they are not used to such an intense backbend while resting on the knees. Before trying the posture on a normal surface, have a go at it while kneeling on the mattress in your bedroom. The extra cushion will allow you move back into the Camel with far less stress on the thighs and lower back, and will give you some indication of how simple or challenging the full Camel may be for you. If you find it impossible even on a mattress, then I recommend you continue practising the other backbends for a while before returning to the Camel.

1. Begin by kneeling, with the tops of the feet on the ground, the arms at the sides of the body and the spine erect. The knees and feet should be together, but if this is uncomfortable, separate them slightly.

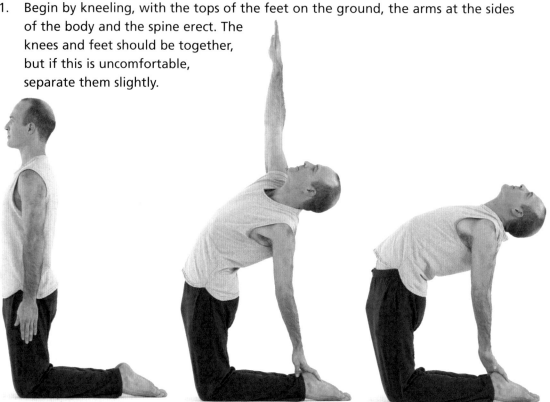

2. Take the right arm overhead and slowly lean backwards, arching the spine until that point where the breathing starts to become constricted, at the same time gently pressing the pelvic area forward. At this point slowly reach down with the left arm to the left heel, keeping the right arm extended upward.
3. Rest the hands or fingers on the heel of the left foot, palm facing towards the buttocks.
4. When the left hand is resting comfortably, then slowly lower the right hand down to the right heel.
5. Push the pelvic area and abdomen forward, trying to touch an imaginary wall in front of you with your abdomen. Open the tops of the shoulders out and back, trying to squeeze the shoulder blades together. Allow the chin to stretch up towards the sky. Breathe normally and try to relax the body into the stretch.

Beginner's variation: Camel on High Heels
If it is too much for the tops of your feet to be flat on the ground, then tuck the toes under and rest on the balls of the feet with the heels pointing up instead. For beginners this may be especially helpful as it also raises the heel and makes it easier to rest the hands there.

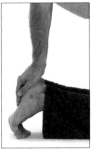

6. While in the posture the weight of the body should be evenly distributed through the legs and arms.
7. To come out of the posture, release the pelvis and abdomen back down, then raise the torso by pressing the right arm down on the heel and straightening the body slowly while reaching the other arm up – this lifts the body without putting any strain on the back.

The stretch on the front of the body and thighs while in the Camel is extreme, but you should always be aware of the lower back in the posture. As other parts of the body ache, it is easy to forget that this is a backbending posture and to sag the body in order to relieve the strain, thereby compressing the spine. Keep the front of the body extending forward and up all the time.

Benefits: The Camel is beneficial for digestive and reproductive systems. It stretches the stomach and intestines, alleviating constipation. It relieves stiffness in the vertebrae and stimulates spinal nerves, relieving backache, lumbago and a rounded back. The front of the neck is stretched, stimulating the thyroid.

Common mistakes: Too often people fall backwards instead of arching into the stretch, putting stress on the lower back. Forward pressure through the abdomen should be maintained. The shoulders should not hunch forward, but should extend away from the ears and drop down and back. Do not allow the head to drop too far back, but tilt the chin up and ensure breathing remains comfortable throughout.

Contraindications: People with severe back problems should not try this posture without proper guidance.

Sequence: Ideally during backbending, and when the body is warm so your spine is prepared, so long as a mild forward stretch of the spine in the opposite direction is attempted immediately afterwards. Such a counterpose should be light and passive, such as Child's Pose or extended Cat postures.

Awareness: Physical – on the abdomen, throat, spine or breathing. Energetic – swadhisthana or vishuddhi chakra.

Cat (Bidalasana)
Level: 1

I'm sure you have seen a cat arch its back in what looks to be a delicious and fulfilling stretch. Well, the cat knows what it is doing – giving the spine a lovely extension and stretch. It is exactly that principle that you will follow when practising the Cat posture. Enjoy this posture and take your time. Feel the spine stretch and lengthen and open. Use the breathing to go further and further into the movement.

1. Begin on all fours with the wrists directly below the shoulders and the knees directly below the hips. It is vital that both the forearms and the thighs are perpendicular to the ground and remain that way throughout. Relax the body.

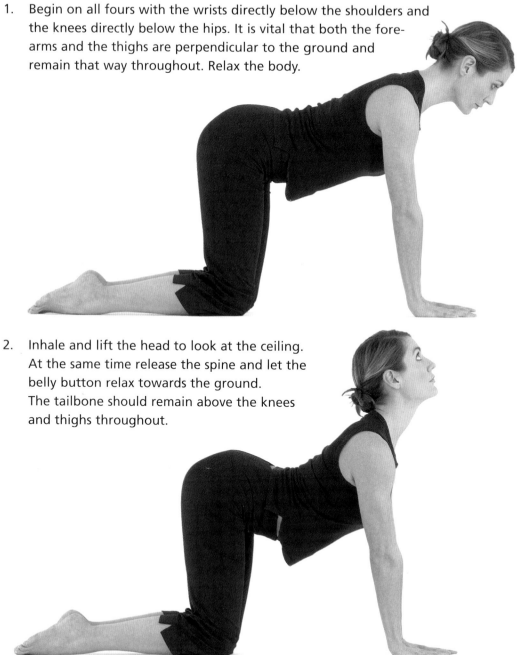

2. Inhale and lift the head to look at the ceiling. At the same time release the spine and let the belly button relax towards the ground. The tailbone should remain above the knees and thighs throughout.

3. Exhale and lower the head all the way so that you are looking through the arms towards the groin area – feel the back of the neck stretch. Lift the spine upward, creating an arch, without rocking forward or backwards on the hands and knees. The spine and the muscles in the back should feel stretched.

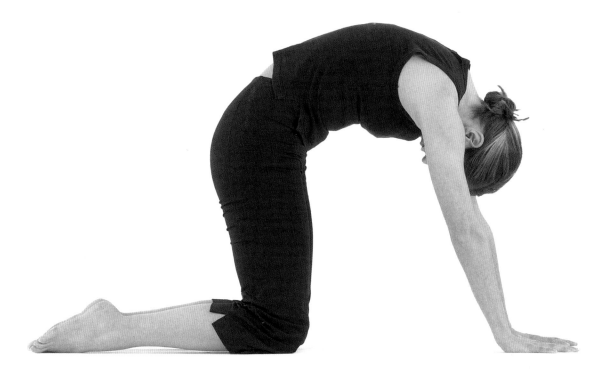

4. Repeat this movement up to 10–15 times in slow rhythmic breaths, focusing on the movement and the stretch of the spinal column with each inhalation and exhalation.

Benefits: Improves flexibility of neck, shoulders and spine. Tones the female reproductive system.

Common mistakes: People often bend the elbows, especially when inhaling. Keep the arms straight throughout. Alignment is vital in the Cat in order to concentrate the stretch on the spine. Do not make sudden movements, but flow through each movement using the breathing as a guide.

Contraindications: None.

Sequence: At the beginning of a practice, to warm up the spine and start to coordinate breath and movement.

Awareness: Physical – coordinating the breathing with movement and the flexion of the spine. Energetic – swadhisthana chakra.

Bridge (Setu Bandhasana)
Level: 1

In the final Bridge position your body should be strong enough so that someone could use you literally as a bridge to cross a stream – at least, that is the theory. What is important is to visualize that kind of strength in the posture, especially in the centre of the bridge where the stress on the structure is at its greatest and where it is easy to allow the body to drop slightly.

1. Lie flat on your back with the knees bent and the feet flat on the ground – the heels should be relatively close to the buttocks. The feet and knees should be together, though for beginners it may be an idea to separate them slightly, hip-width. The arms are close to the side of the body, palms down and flat, fingers slightly spread.

2. Breathing normally, apply pressure through the feet and, moving the knees directly away from you, tilt the pubic bone towards the navel, which will lift the tailbone slightly off the ground. Try to visualize your spine as a string of pearls and as you go up you are peeling each pearl (vertebra) one by one slowly off the ground until the entire lower and middle back and ribcage is lifted. You are now in half Bridge, with the shoulders, knees and hips in one straight diagonal line. As a beginner you could stay in this pose and breathe normally, eventually coming down one vertebra at a time, just as you went up.

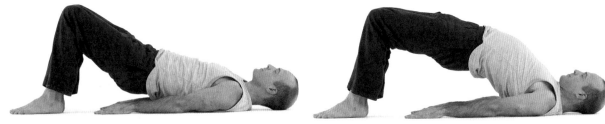

3. If you would like to try the full Bridge, continue moving the knees away from you, pressing down through the shoulders and arms and hands so that the upper back begins to lift from the ground as well. Feel each vertebra lift from the ground one by one. Eventually only the back of your head, neck, shoulders, arms and hands, and of course the feet, should remain on the ground.

4. Lift the chest and abdomen upwards and press the shoulders down and back, opening the chest further. The arms should be straight along the ground, palms down, fingers pointing towards the heels or you could inch the arms under the belly and then place the full palm into the back for a variation on the full bridge. Keep the elbows tucked under the body.

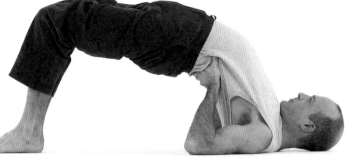

Continue to press the knees away. Hold the position and breathe normally, continually checking to ensure that the chest, abdomen and pelvic area are lifting up.

5. When you are ready to release the posture, slowly lower the chest and abdomen down so that the shoulder blades open away from each other and the upper part of the spine comes back into contact with the ground. Keeping the knees and thighs active, slowly roll the spine back onto the ground one vertebra at a time – remember that string of pearls. Finally rest the tailbone on the ground and relax.

All of the advanced variations to the Bridge that follow are to be attempted only once you are comfortable in the basic Bridge.

Shoulder Pose (Kandharasana)

1. From the Bridge step the feet closer to the buttocks so that you are able to reach down and take hold of each ankle with the hands, palms facing each other. Adjust the body so that the shoulders are fully in contact with the ground, and continue to press away with the knees, simulating the effect and position of the Bow but this time in the opposite direction.

2. Work the shoulder blades together by pressing the shoulders back and down, opening the ribs and chest to promote deep breathing. Press the knees away and create resistance down through the feet with the ground to create an opposing movement so that space is created to push the abdomen higher and deepen the stretch in the lower back.

3. Hold this pose for as long as is comfortable, breathing normally. When you are finished, let go of the ankles and step the feet back to the original starting position. Then slowly lower the body as you would for the original Bridge.

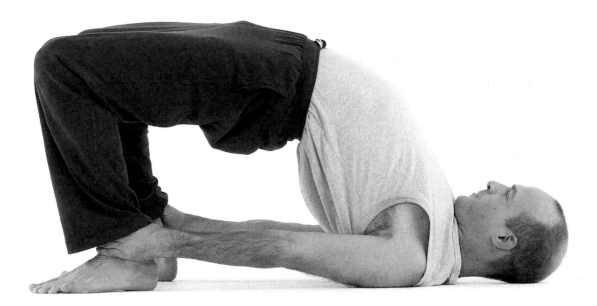

Leg Raises

1. Relax the body as much as possible in the final Bridge position. Inhale, press down through the left foot and lift the right leg off the ground. Straighten the right leg towards the sky and push through the heel of the right foot in order to straighten the leg as much as possible. Press down through the arms and hands to assist you further into the pose; you could also do this variation supporting your back with your hands, fingers towards your spine, thumbs around your torso. Hold the posture for a complete breath.

2. On the next exhalation slowly lower the right leg and return it to the ground.

3. Inhale and repeat to the other side. Repeat both sides 3–5 times.

Passive Backward Bend With Support

In order to remain in the posture for long periods of time and deepen the stretch, many students enjoy placing a block under the back during the Bridge and simply relaxing onto it for as long as it is comfortable, which, if the block is placed correctly, can often be a very long time.

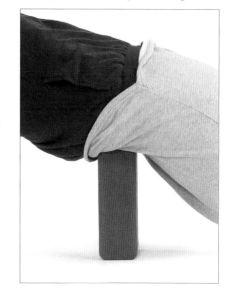

Have the block next to you within easy reaching distance when you begin moving up into the basic Bridge. When you are in the complete Bridge reach for the block and place it under the lower part of the spine. Whether you place the block lengthways or widthways up depends on how deeply you can move into the basic Bridge and how high the abdomen is lifted during the posture.

As you can see from the picture, the block should be placed at the bottom of the spine, just above the sacrum, in a natural groove that you should find quite easily in your own back. The sacrum is a flat pear-shaped bone above the last vertebra, the tailbone. When placed correctly, the lower back should feel very comfortable with no stress on it. Remain in this position for as long as is comfortable, breathing freely.

Benefits: This posture is excellent for realignment of the spine, eliminating rounded shoulders and relieving backache. It massages the colon and abdominal organs, improving digestion. It tones the female reproductive system.

Common mistakes: The knees and legs have a natural tendency to flare apart to the sides. Keep your knees above your feet; it may help to hold a block between the knees to stop them releasing outwards. Also, keep the feet flat on the ground. Do not allow the abdomen to drop, but use the upward movement of the chest and abdomen to continually lift the torso towards the sky, ensuring that the spine remains arched and fully stretched throughout. The shoulders, arms and hands should press back and down throughout so that the upper part of the spine does not collapse onto the ground. Keep the back of the neck extended and flat on the ground, chin towards the chest.

Contraindications: Anyone suffering from abdominal hernia should not practise this posture. It is recommended that pregnant women should avoid the full Bridge completely.

Sequence: The Bridge may be used at various points in your practice:
a. As part of a general backbending sequence and when the body and spine are warm from previous postures.
b. As a link between the Shoulderstand and the Fish (explained in the Inverted section).
c. As preparation for the Wheel.
d. Before a forward bending posture.

Awareness: Physical – on the movement, the abdominal area, the thyroid gland or flexion of the back. Energetic – on vishuddhi or anahata chakra.

Wheel (Chakrasana)
Level: 3

This is one of those postures that as children we could probably do with ease. Gradually as we age our spinal column stiffens and movements such as the Wheel can become a real challenge. Although the Wheel is a demanding pose in terms of strength and flexibility, it can be assisted and made much simpler if you remember to lift the heart throughout. Be sure to be properly warmed up before attempting it, and don't be discouraged if at first you cannot even lift yourself fractionally off the ground. It takes time, so be patient and just keep trying.

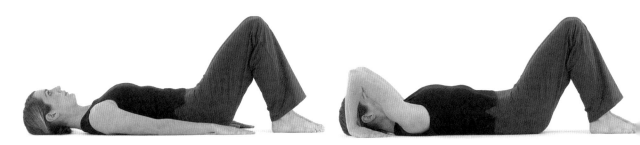

1. Lie flat on the back with the knees bent and the feet flat on the ground. The heels should be relatively close to the buttocks. The feet and knees should be hip-width apart. The arms should be resting down alongside the body, palms down.
2. Bend the elbows and take the arms behind you so the palms are flat on the floor by the ears.

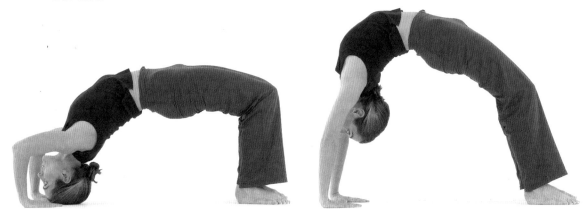

3. Lift the heart and press down through the buttocks, creating a lift in the lower back. As the heart lifts, continue to press the shoulders down and away, so that the shoulder blades squeeze together. Adjust the hands to ensure they are flat on the ground and the fingertips are just under the top of the shoulders. Exhale and place the crown of the head on the floor, creating a mini wheel. You may want to practice this for a while until you feel you have the body strength to continue into the full wheel.

To continue, exhale and push through the hands and feet to lift the torso higher, leading with the heart to the sky. Try to straighten the arms completely. Press the knees up and away, lifting the thighs and imagining your pelvis reaching towards the sky. Visualize a string attached to your belly button, lifting you upward.

Advanced Variation:
Straighten the legs, lift up through the heart and allow the head to hang freely between the arms. Breathe! To come down follow step 7.

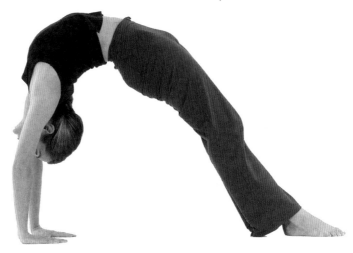

6. Hold the final position for as long as is comfortable, breathing normally.
7. Slowly lower the body with control so that first the head rests on the floor, as in stage 3, then lower the buttocks and finally tuck the tailbone in to lower the spine.

Benefits: The Wheel is beneficial to the nervous, digestive, respiratory, cardiovascular and glandular systems. It tones the arms and legs and reduces excess fat around the waistline.

Common mistakes: The Wheel is very much a strength posture, and therefore most mistakes are caused by people simply not being strong enough to lift up into the full posture. Keep the thighs rotating inwards, which will keep the knees over the feet, and avoid compression of the lower back, creating space to arch into the pose further.

Contraindications: Should not be practised during any times of illness or pregnancy. Those with especially weak wrists should not attempt until strengthening work has been done.

Sequence: The Wheel should not be attempted until the other backbending postures have been practised and the spine is flexible and shoulders strong. Once that is the case it can be part of a normal backbending sequence or done after the Bridge.

Awareness: Physical – on relaxation of the spine and opening of the chest and abdomen. Energetic – on manipura chakra.

Lying Spinal Twist Cycle

The backbending postures are intense stretches of the spine that are often among the most demanding for beginners. After a sequence of backbending postures it is always advisable as a counterpose to do some side-to-side twisting and rotation of the spine in order to flex the vertebral discs and straighten the spine. After twisting the body you may then continue with your next sequence of postures. The first should include some sort of forward bend to bring the spine back to a neutral alignment. The twists given here are very simple ones that should give a relaxing rotation to the spine. I have given the benefits, common mistakes, contraindications, sequencing and awareness at the end of all the twisting postures, on page 127, as they are the same for all twists.

Double Knee Spinal Twist
Level: 1

1. Begin lying flat on your back. Bend the knees and lift the feet off the ground so that the shins are parallel to the floor. Stretch your arms out to both sides of the body.
2. Keeping the knees and feet together, exhale and allow both knees to release to the ground to the side. Take the knees as far as they will go, but do not force them to the ground. Allow the hips to rotate and the top buttock to lift from the ground as you twist. Look to the opposite side.
3. Inhale and bring the knees and head back to centre.
4. Exhale and repeat to the other side.
5. Continue to move to each side in time with the breathing. Repeat up to 10 times for each side. If you wish to relax to one side for longer periods, feel free to do so as long as you go down on an exhalation and come back to centre on an inhalation.

Advanced variation
To deepen the stretch and strengthen the body try straight-ening the legs above you in step 1 and then repeating the movement to each side, remembering the breathing, with legs straight and together. It may be easier to hold this posture for longer periods on each side and then bend the knees to the centre.

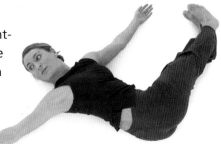

124

Lying Eagle Spinal Twist
Level: 1

1. Begin lying flat on your back. Bend the knees and lift the feet off the ground so that the shins are parallel to the floor. Stretch your arms out to both sides of the body, palms down.

2. Bring the right leg over the left leg and try to hook your right foot round the back of the left calf.

3. Keeping the legs in Eagle position, exhale and allow both knees to release to the ground to the left-hand side. Take the knees as far as they will go, but do not

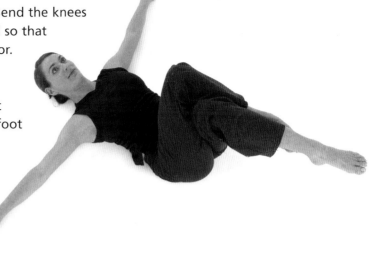

force them to the ground. Allow the hips to rotate and the right buttock to lift from the ground as you twist. Look to the right-hand side.

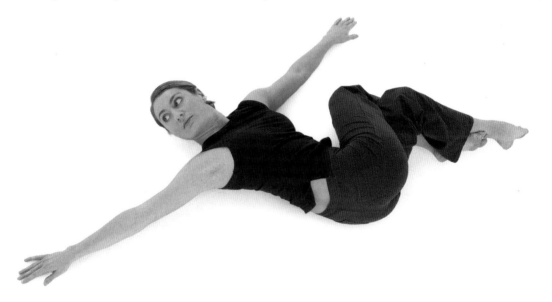

4. Inhale and bring the knees and head back to centre.

5. Exhale and repeat to the other side, changing the twist of the legs, so the left leg comes over the right leg and hooks round the right calf.

6. If you wish to relax to each side for longer periods, feel free to do so, breathing naturally, as long as you go down on an exhalation and come back to centre on an inhalation.

Single Leg Spinal Twists
Level: 1

1. Begin lying flat on your back. Bend the knees and lift the feet off the ground so that the shins are parallel to the floor.
2. Place your hands on your knees and allow the weight of your hands and arms to press the knees towards the chest. Relax and feel the spine lengthen.
3. Straighten your left leg out along the ground, feeling the buttocks press into the ground and the heel pull away.
4. Place the left hand on top of your right kneecap. Place your right arm along the ground at a slight diagonal going upwards and away from the right ear with the palm up.

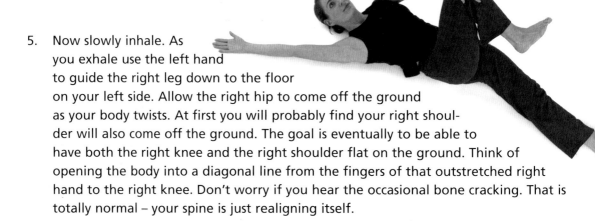

5. Now slowly inhale. As you exhale use the left hand to guide the right leg down to the floor on your left side. Allow the right hip to come off the ground as your body twists. At first you will probably find your right shoulder will also come off the ground. The goal is eventually to be able to have both the right knee and the right shoulder flat on the ground. Think of opening the body into a diagonal line from the fingers of that outstretched right hand to the right knee. Don't worry if you hear the occasional bone cracking. That is totally normal – your spine is just realigning itself.

6. When you are in the posture try to relax as much as possible, using the exhalation to soften and relax the shoulders and to sink into the spiral your body has created. Always think of lengthening the spine.

7. Stay here for 3–6 long, deep breaths. Then bring the right knee back to the chest and bend the left leg back towards your chest.

8. Repeat the twist to the other side, with the right hand leading the left leg down to the ground.

Advanced variation

Follow the above sequence all the way to step 5, then straighten the leg out along the ground, trying to take hold of the leg where comfortable. Eventually the aim could be to hold the toes. Remain in this pose for as long as comfortable, breathing normally. When you are ready to come out of the posture, bend the knee back to where you started and continue following the steps above. Repeat on the other leg.

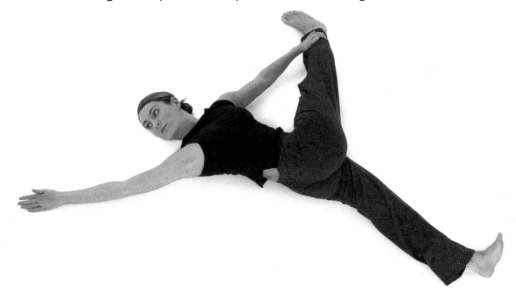

Benefits: The postures in this sequence relieve tiredness and tightness, especially in the lower back. Pelvic and abdominal organs are squeezed through the massaging action of the twist. Rectifies disorders of the hip joints. Excellent for people who sit for long periods. Stimulates the nervous system. Improves digestion and eliminates constipation. Helps keep the spine mobile through rotation.

Common mistakes: Arms and hands not pressing down into the floor. The opposite shoulder to the rotation lifts too much from the floor. Holding the breath.

Contraindications: People with lower back problems should approach with caution.

Sequence: After backbending postures, as a warm-up, or during a floor sequence (sitting postures).

Awareness: Physical – on length and rotation. Energetic – on manipura chakra.

Inverted Postures

Inspiration is in every breath

Anon

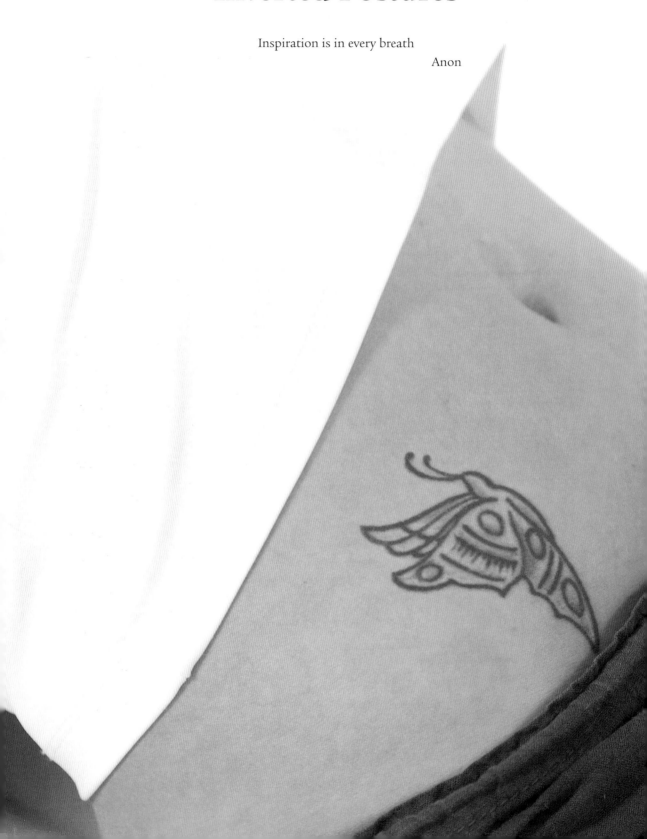

Inverted postures reverse the action of gravity on the body, allowing us to touch the ground with the head and allowing energy to flow through the body in the opposite direction to what is the case 99.9 per cent of our lives. The postures increase health, reduce anxiety and stress, and do wonders to our confidence by enabling us to face up directly to the fears we carry around with us all the time. For this reason yoga practitioners hold inverted postures in the highest possible regard, and the Headstand and Shoulderstand are considered the king and queen of yoga postures, respectively.

Inverted postures encourage a fresh supply of blood to rush to the brain, nourishing the neurons and flushing out toxins. The circulation of blood is reversed, purifying and energizing the entire body. This process nourishes the cells of the entire body, enriching the blood flow and tuning the endocrine system. All of this has a positive effect on the metabolic system and on your mental state.

Inverted postures are also among the most demanding of all yoga postures. They take time, patience and complete awareness as you enter, maintain and come out of the pose. In fact, this is the case with all postures. To assist you, there are a few guidelines that you should follow whenever you try inverted postures.

1. Never practise inverted postures or any poses immediately after a meal. You are going upside down, so please give yourself a few hours after you have eaten before you practise. Neither should you practise inverted postures when you are tired. This point may seem less obvious. Inverted postures are extremely demanding, especially for beginners, so I recommend that you practise these postures at the beginning of a session after your Sun Salutations or when the body is warm enough and your energy is at its highest level.

2. Do not overexert yourself in the postures. Beginners should stay for only a matter of seconds in the final positions to enable them to come out of the pose with grace, and only once the posture can be maintained without experiencing the slightest difficulty should the length of the posture be extended.

3. Be sure to practise inverted postures in a clear space. If you do lose your balance during an inverted posture, which is quite normal to begin with, it is much better to fall out completely of the posture in a relaxed state than it is to have a piece of furniture, for instance, block your fall halfway down.

4. Always follow inverted postures with a period of rest. I will suggest some of the best resting positions for each pose, as well as giving the counterbalances that are important to ensure your body is getting a complete stretch in every direction.

5. Many schools of thought say that women should not practise inverted postures when they have their period, as it goes against the natural energy flow of the body. I would strongly agree with this but, as with so many other aspects of yoga, you are the best judge of whether or not it is right for you.

I have divided the inverted postures into three broad sections: Headstand and variations, Shoulderstand and variations, and finally Handstand and variations. Many variations involve using a wall to assist you in the posture. Try not to get too comfortable with using walls. As soon as you feel confident, move away from them and try the postures freestanding. Inverted postures are truly special. I hope you enjoy them as much as do. However, please make sure to take care.

The Dolphin
Level: 1

In this section I will start by explaining the Dolphin. The Dolphin can be of great assistance in building body strength to lift up into the inverted postures, especially through the shoulders. Once you are proficient in the inverted postures there is no more need to practise the Dolphin, although as an exercise to strengthen the shoulders it is highly effective and recommended

1. Begin in a kneeling position. Take each palm to the opposite elbow, and then bring your arms forward to the ground in front of you a comfortable distance away from the body. Move your hands away from the elbows, without the elbows moving from their spot on the ground at all, interlock your fingers and put your hands into a fist in front of you. Look at a point just in front of the interlocked hands and relax the body. Ensure that the knees are underneath the hips and elbows under the shoulders.

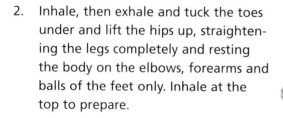

2. Inhale, then exhale and tuck the toes under and lift the hips up, straightening the legs completely and resting the body on the elbows, forearms and balls of the feet only. Inhale at the top to prepare.

3. Exhale, bring the weight forward so that the head comes forward of the hands, with the chin almost touching the ground in front of you. Keep the spine and legs straight throughout and the abdomen muscles engaged.

4. Inhale, press down through the elbows, push the shoulders down and lift the hips back up to the starting position. Repeat 10–15 times, or build up to what is comfortable in your body, remembering it's not the quantity you do but the quality that matters. Use the breath as your guide and try to keep the movements slow and steady.

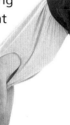

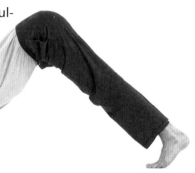

A simpler variation

It is also possible to practise Dolphin with the knees on the ground if the body does not have the strength for the full variation just yet. In this case you would begin the practice in the position described in step 1 above, and then simply move forward and back as in steps 3 and 4 above, with the knees remaining in contact with the ground throughout. It is important to keep the abdominal muscles engaged to prevent your spine from overarching.

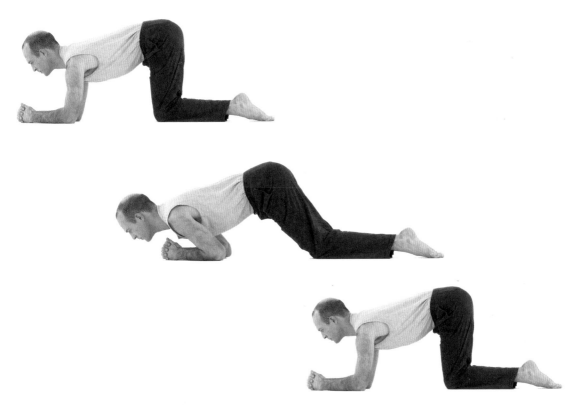

Benefits: Strengthens the upper body in preparation for headstand and inverted postures.

Mistakes: Not contracting the abdominal muscles, allowing the spine to overarch and collapse. In the full version, allowing the legs to bend. They should remain straight throughout.

Contraindications: If you have any shoulder problems approach with caution.

Sequence: After Sun Salutation when the body is warm. Before inversions to prepare the body for them.

Awareness: Physical – on maintaining the strength in the abdominal muscles and creating a rhythm with the movement and breath. Energetic – on manipura chakra.

Headstand

The Headstand (sirsasana) is the king of yoga postures. Although it is of course a challenging posture to learn, it is often the case that beginners make it harder than it actually is. A great amount of fear and doubt can be involved in learning the Headstand. Often the act of practising the Headstand is as much about overcoming mental blocks as it is physical limitations.

For those who have a fear of inverting the body it is possible to practise the Headstand against a wall. However, I do not recommend using the wall for your entire means of support as this can lead to dependence on it. Instead I recommend that you practise the posture just in front of the wall, giving yourself about 3–5 inches from the front of the hands below to the bottom of the wall. This is close enough to prevent you from toppling over, a common fear, yet far enough away to allow you to properly practise the Headstand without assistance.

It is remarkable how many students, once they are actually in the Headstand, say how much easier it is than they originally thought.

The Headstand (Sirsanana)
Level: 2–3

There are eight steps to Headstand. (And two steps to come out again.) Visualize yourself as eight building blocks, which you place one directly on top of the other as you go up – so you need to build a firm foundation from the bottom up. Take your time with each step, being aware of every movement you make, and keeping your breath rhythmical and steady to stay focused. Enjoy.
Begin in a kneeling position, spine erect and hands on either thigh. Relax and breathe comfortably for a few moments.

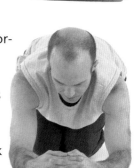

1.   Then fold one arm over the other and hold each elbow. Bend forward and place the forearms on the ground a comfortable distance away from the body. Do not allow the elbows to move from this position during the pose. The elbows act as two-thirds of the tripod that is needed to effectively balance your Headstand.

2.   Release the hands from the elbows in front of you and interlock the fingers, without moving the elbows, so that the palms form a cup. Lock the fingers well, as your head will rest and balance in the cup the palms form. (Note: many different hand positions may be used in the Headstand and the one I am describing here is simply the most common. Experiment with different hand positions – for instance, a fist – but remember the vital thing is that the hands form a secure cup for the head to rest in during the Headstand.)

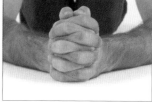

3. Rest the top of the head on the ground between the interlocked fingers so that the back of the head touches the cupped palms. Do not rest the forehead or the back of the head on the ground. What is important is to keep the length at the back of the neck.

4. After securing a comfortable head and neck position, gently press the shoulders away from the ears and engage the abdomen muscles. On an exhalation, tuck the toes under and lift the buttocks, straightening the legs in the process. Keep lifting the buttocks to ensure your spine is as straight as possible. At this point, gravity will want to take you down, and you need to resist that feeling by lifting up. Visualize balloons attached to your buttocks lifting you up. You are now in half a Headstand where you could stay, still gaining part of the benefits.

5. Walk the feet in towards the head in small steps as far as you can go, trying to make sure that your spine does not buckle. Keep pressing the shoulders away from the ears and feeling your arms resisting the floor to encourage your spine to elongate. When you approach the limit that you can walk towards the head, you should feel upward pressure on your feet, as if they are trying to leave the ground. If you cannot feel this pressure, then continue to lift the buttocks higher and try to walk the feet in further towards the head. Try to get to the point where your hips are directly above your shoulders before you continue to the next step. Remember those building blocks one on top of the other, hips above shoulders.

6. Push both feet off the ground gently and lift the knees in towards the abdomen, trying to straighten the spine by lifting the buttocks towards the sky and pushing down through the shoulders. It is this stage that beginners find the most challenging, simply because it is hard to see your own spine straighten and lift up as the feet leave the ground. However, if you can do this step, then the rest of the Headstand is relatively simple in comparison.

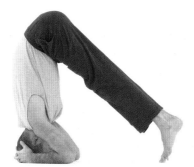

Beginner's variation to step 6

Those who are uncomfortable lifting both feet off the ground at once, try to bring one foot off the ground at a time. To do this walk the feet in towards the body as much as possible as in step 5 and then lift one foot off the ground and bend the knee in towards the abdomen. Focus on lifting the buttocks and straightening the spine in order that the other foot rises onto the tips of the toes and begins to feel additional pressure to lift. Try this on the other side. When you are ready, simply try to lift the foot off the ground as in step 5. Do not try to push up into the full Headstand immediately. Instead focus on trying to maintain balance at this point, pressing the shoulders away from the ears and pressing the buttocks up in order to lengthen the spine. Touch your feet together, so you have a sense of where you are upside down. Keep engaging the abdomen muscles and breathe deeply.

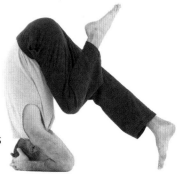

7. Lift the knees slowly straight up into the air, keeping them bent. The heels should come back towards the buttocks. In doing so you come into the three-quarters Headstand, with only the lower half of the legs to extend. It is vital to take your time over this movement. Keep the abdomen muscles engaged and breathe steadily throughout.

8. Straighten out the legs above you, pull up through the heels, engaging your buttocks and abdomen, and push down through the shoulders to straighten the body. Breathe normally and work at relaxing the body. It would be helpful if you asked a friend to check your alignment and ensure that you are straight from the shoulders to the heels. Many beginners use their pelvic area to lever themselves into a place where they feel balanced, but often this causes them to bring the legs forward to counterbalance the pelvis pushing back. When you are properly straight it may feel quite unbalanced at first, but this is simply due to your body's inexperience of being inverted. You are now in a full Headstand.

9. Stay as long in the Headstand as is comfortable, maybe starting with 5 breaths in the pose, and adding rounds of breath each time you practice so you can measure your progress. The moment you feel any strain in the body, begin coming out of the posture by reversing the steps that you took coming into the posture. First, bend the knees so that the heels come down by the buttocks as in step 7. Then bring your knees into your chest as in step 6 and straighten the legs out and allow them to release slowly to the ground. It is essential that you take your time coming out of the Headstand, and it is for this reason that I would never advise staying in the posture as long as you possibly can until your entire body is shaking and you have no strength to come out of it comfortably.

10. When your feet are back on the ground, release down to your knees and relax in Child's Pose for at least 5 long relaxed breaths. This will balance the blood flow in the body and prevent any dizziness.

For those who wish to practise against a wall the best place to practise is positioned diagonally in the corner so that you are protected from falling sideways. It is sometimes recommended that you actually practise toppling over out of a Headstand in order to dispel that particular fear. The key is to bend the knees and tuck the head in so that the natural arch of the spine rolls you safely onto the ground. Once you see that very little harm can come from the Headstand so long as the body is relaxed, many of your fears should disappear.

Benefits: Regular practice makes healthy pure blood flow through the brain cells, encouraging clear thinking. This flow of blood also washes over the pineal and pituitary glands, ensuring proper functioning of these important glands for health, growth and vitality. Due to gravity being reversed on the spine, strain on the back is alleviated and tissue regeneration in the legs is encouraged. The weight of the abdominal organs on the diaphragm encourages deep breathing, expelling toxins from the system. Regular practice develops the body and calms the mind. The heart has a rest in the inverted position. Digestive organs are massaged. Circulation is improved. The back and shoulders are strengthened.

Common mistakes: The most obvious mistake in Headstand is incorrect alignment of the body. Balance alone is not enough: you must constantly be aware of the subtle movements of the body. The weight of the body should be taken by the head, although the arms should act as support. Do not allow the shoulders to sag down towards the ground, but continually push them away from the ears. When in the full Headstand the legs should not be allowed to bend: keep them together and push up through the heels. The elbows act as two points of the tripod that will maintain your balance in the posture, so ensure that they do not drift apart.

Contraindications: Some say that anyone with high blood pressure, heart disease, thrombosis, constipation, kidney problems, conjunctivitis, glaucoma and many other diseases should not practise the Headstand. However, there are also those who say that regular practice will assist in the prevention and cure of all those, and many other, ailments. If you have any serious health problems, discuss with your doctor the potential benefits or harm of practising this posture.

Sequence: Beginners should practise the Headstand towards the beginning of their session, after properly warming up, because of the effort involved in the posture. The placing of the Headstand is not as important for proficient students, so long as it is followed by Shoulderstand or another counterpose such as Child's Pose.

Awareness: Physical – for beginners on maintaining balance. For advanced students on the brain, centre of the head or breathing. Energetic – on sahasrara chakra.

Advanced Variation

This variation to the Headstand should not be attempted until you are confident and comfortable with the basic Headstand, although for some this will feel simpler.

Supported Headstand (Salamba Sirsasana)
Level: 3

The Supported Headstand is similar to the basic Headstand with one main difference: instead of the elbows forming two of the bases of the supporting tripod, the palms this time are the supports, with the elbows lifted and the upper arms parallel to the ground. In this variation you will feel much more weight through the arms, but you should avoid the temptation to allow all the weight to go through the hands, as this will result in improper balance. The head should still take a large amount of the weight, with the hands serving primarily a balancing function.

1. Begin on all fours with the hands directly below the shoulders, fingers spread and pointing forward, and the knees below the hips.
2. Bend the elbows and bring the head forward to rest on the ground. The area between the crown and forehead should be in contact with the ground. Slide the hands slightly back so that a triangle is formed between the hands and the head. Begin to press down through the palms. Tuck the toes under.
3. Lift the buttocks and straighten the legs so that only the head, hands and toes are in contact with the ground. At this point you should ensure that your hands are pressing firmly into the ground and that the head is in a comfortable position on the ground. Walk the feet in towards the head as much as possible. Follow the same principles as in the Headstand as to the shape of the spine.
4. Push both feet off the ground gently and lift the knees in towards the abdomen, trying to straighten the spine by lifting the buttocks upwards and pushing down through the hands.

5. Lift the knees straight up into the air, keeping the knees bent. The heels should be moving towards the buttocks.

6. Straighten out the legs above you, pull up through the heels, which will engage the buttocks, firm the abdomen and push down through the hands to straighten the body. Breathe normally and work at relaxing the body. Check your alignment at this point. The tendency is for the body to begin to fall back towards the ground as weight is pushed onto the hands and arms. Keep lifting the legs and straightening the body.

7. Stay in the Supported Headstand as long as is comfortable. The moment you feel any strain in the body, begin coming out of the posture by reversing the steps you took coming into it. First, bend the knees so that the heels come down by the buttocks. Then bring the knees in towards the chest and straighten the legs out and allow them to release slowly to the ground.

8. When your feet are back on the ground, relax down to your knees and rest in Child's Pose for at least 5 long relaxed breaths. This is in order to balance the blood flow in the body and prevent any dizziness that might be caused by coming back up to a normal sitting or standing position too quickly.

Benefits, etc: As for the basic Headstand.

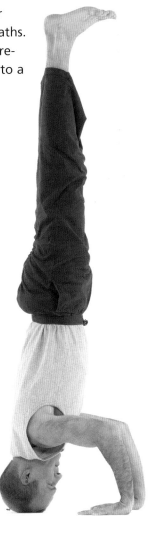

Scorpion (Vrschikasana)
Level: 3

The scorpion is a very advanced Headstand variation and can be a daunting postures for any student to master. In most cases, mastery is as much mental as physical. The Scorpion is a supreme test of balance, strength and body awareness. There are many ways in which the scorpion is taught, and I will show the way from the basic Headstand. Many people find that practising the Scorpion near a wall is beneficial, as the wall acts as something for the feet to rest against, minimizing the fear of toppling over.

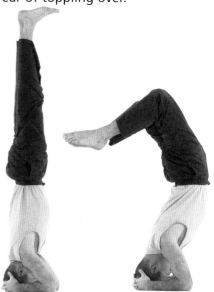

1. Make your way into the basic Headstand. Relax the body and breathe normally.

2. Slowly arch the back so that the abdomen moves forward – keeping it engaged gently will keep your centre strong. As you do this, begin to bend the knees so that the feet release towards the ground behind your head. Go only as far as is comfortable, and try to find a point of balance where the forward movement of the abdomen acts as a natural counterweight to the backward movement of the feet. Visualize a pendulum. It is vital that this point of balance is found for the rest of the posture to be attempted. It is often helpful to touch the toes together so you can get an understanding of where your legs and feet are.

Beginner's variation

If you wish to practise the Scorpion against the wall, which many beginners prefer, then set up in your normal Headstand approximately a foot away from the wall. By creating this distance you allow your feet to come over your body sufficiently to enter the Scorpion while resting your toes against a wall and minimizing the risk of falling. To exit follow step 6.

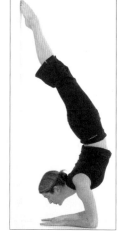

3. After securing the balance, move the forearms carefully, without moving the elbows, so that the hands lie either side of the head, parallel to each other, palms flat on the floor, fingers spread. Once again ensure you are properly balanced before proceeding.

4. Slowly raise the head from the ground and look forward as much as possible, lifting the heart so that you are balancing on your forearms only. Lift up through the arms and shoulders so that the upper arms are as vertical as possible.

5. Try to relax the whole body as much you can, finding a spot to focus on. Hold for as long as is comfortable, breathing normally.

6. To exit the Scorpion, lower the head slowly towards the ground and replace the hands behind the head, interlocking the fingers as in the basic Headstand pose. Then simultaneously bring the knees towards the chest and straighten the back, using the abdomen muscles to aid this action. This takes you into the three-quarters Headstand, and you should come out of this pose as explained on page 134.

Advanced variation

From step 4, try to straighten the legs above you. This will test your balance and strength so be very careful. Keep the abdominal muscles engaged. To exit this Scorpion follow step 6 above.

Benefits: The Scorpion increases the blood flow to the brain and pituitary gland, revitalizing the bodily systems. It increases circulation in the lower limbs and abdomen, and tones the reproductive systems. The arched position tones and stretches the back, arms and shoulders.

Common mistakes: The Scorpion is a mental test, and therefore the most common mistake is not bringing enough weight down through the feet, not bringing them near enough to the head, for fear of falling backwards. This would mean never being able to enter the full Scorpion, and is why it may be helpful to practise near a wall at first. The other common mistake is sagging through the shoulders. The shoulders and upper arms should be kept strong and extended throughout. The abdomen muscles should be engaged throughout.

Contraindications: As with Headstand. This posture should never be attempted until the other inverted poses can be done without difficulty.

Sequence: During a sequence of inverted postures. Once the body is warm and strengthened from preparations such as Plank and Dolphin.

Awareness: Physical – on maintaining balance. Energetic – on ajna chakra.

Movement charts for the Headstand, Supported Headstand and Scorpion

As we have seen these are challenging postures, though hugely beneficial. It is important you follow the technique carefully in order to get into and out of the postures safely. The charts on page 140 will give you a quick reminder of the steps.

The Headstand

Getting Into Position

Getting Out of Position

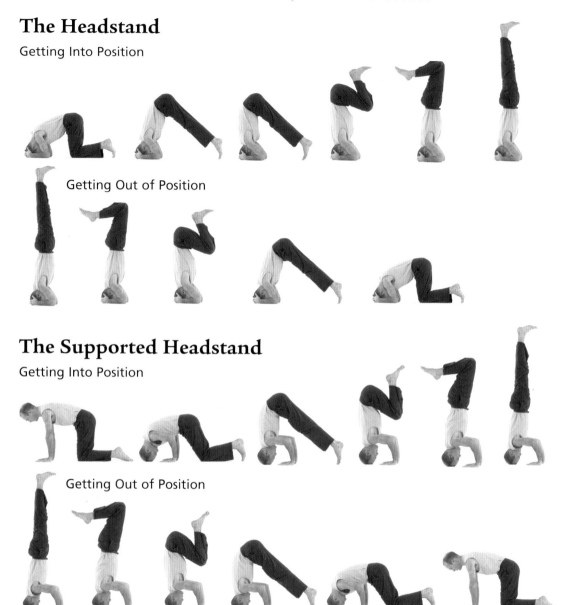

The Supported Headstand

Getting Into Position

Getting Out of Position

The Scorpion

Getting Into Position

Getting Out of Position

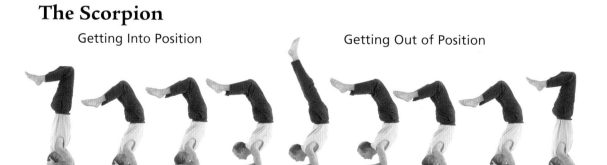

The Shoulderstand Cycle

The Shoulderstand cycle includes the basic Shoulderstand and variations, including variations using a wall, the Plough and its variations, the Fish and its variations, and finally the movement from Shoulderstand into the Bridge position.

The Shoulderstand is a relatively simple posture to do, but a challenging one to master. It involves great strength and flexibility in the upper back and shoulders, and is intended to be held for long periods. Sarvangasana, the Sanskrit name for Shoulderstand, translates as 'all-parts pose' and when you are in the full Shoulderstand it is easy to see why. The Shoulderstand uses virtually all the muscles in the body to some extent. After the Headstand, the Shoulderstand is considered to be the next most beneficial posture. Developing a solid practice of this posture will produce huge benefits to you.

Shoulderstand (Sarvangasana)
Level: 2

I will teach two variations of the Shoulderstand here. The first involves the use of a wall and will assist you in understanding the mechanics of the Shoulderstand. The second is the 'freestanding' or basic Shoulderstand. It is recommended that even those with good flexibility should try the variation using the wall to begin with, simply so that you can feel comfortable in the posture and understand where the pressure points in the body are. As soon as you feel your balance is steady in this version, then you should be ready to move away from the wall and try the basic Shoulderstand. A vital point is not to move your head from side to side.

Beginner's Variation: Shoulderstand with Wall

1. Lie flat on your back with your legs up a wall, keeping a slight bend in the knees, enough to keep the soles of the feet in contact with the wall. Your buttocks should be touching, or very close to, the wall. Place the arms at the side of the body, palms down.

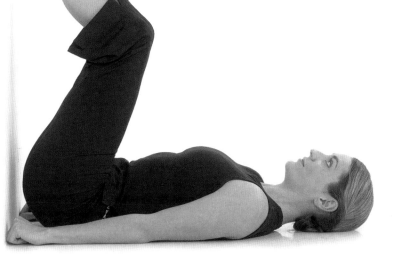

2. Press down through the arms, and press against the wall with the feet, beginning to lift the buttocks off the ground. Slowly lift one vertebra at a time until you have lifted as much of the spine as possible off the ground. The knees should remain bent throughout. Wriggle the shoulders underneath you, trying to bring the shoulder blades together so you now have weight on the shoulders rather than the back of the neck.

3. Lift one arm and place the hand on the ribcage, fingers pointing in towards the spine and thumb around the ribs.

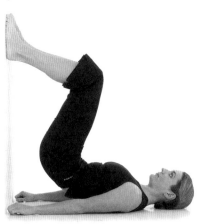 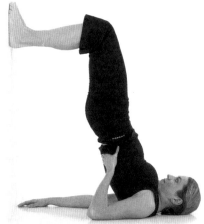

4. Lift the other hand and place it on the other side of the ribcage. Continue to press through the feet and lift the spine. Place both hands against the back ribs to push the chest towards the chin and try to move the spine off the ground so that you are supporting the weight on the arms, nape of the neck, shoulders and back of the head. Don't move your head in the Shoulderstand, just keep on looking up. Try to walk the hands down the back so that your elbows can move in towards each other.

5. Slowly remove the right foot from the wall and straighten

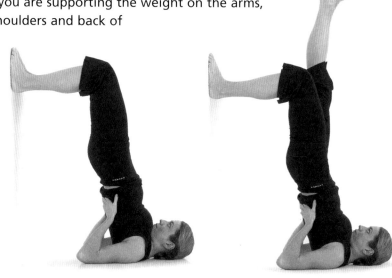

the right leg directly up. Move the sole of the left foot off the wall so that only the toes are in contact with the wall. Examine your balance in this position and see where the stress, if any, in the body occurs. After a few breaths return the right foot to the wall and keep extending the body upward, relaxing as you go.

6. Repeat on the other side, again being aware of the balance and strain this posture puts on the body. Maybe experiment a little bit with your balance by bringing one leg further forward while pushing against the wall with only your toes. Be aware of how your balance changes as the position of the legs changes. After a few breaths return the left foot to the wall and keep extending the body upward, relaxing as you go.

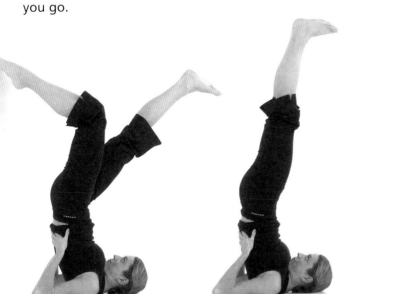

7. If you are comfortable staying up in the pose then continue with this step. (Alternatively, come out of the pose as in step 8 and re-enter the pose when you feel ready.) Moving one foot away from the wall at a time, and keeping a firm base through the arms, try to come into the full Shoulderstand. Once again be aware of the balance and examine how the shifting weight affects your shoulders, arms and head. To help lift you higher up in the Shoulderstand you can cross the ankles, squeeze the buttocks and lift up, walking your hands further down towards your neck. Do make sure you repeat this cross on each side. Try to stay in the full Shoulderstand for a few comfortable breaths. You may find that it is easier to take deep abdominal breaths in the full Shoulderstand. If your balance is not steady then simply return your feet to the wall and continue to experiment with one leg at a time, focusing on your arms, shoulders and head as the foundation of your Shoulderstand.

8. When you are ready to come out of the posture, simply return the feet to the wall. Remove the hands from the back and place them back on the floor alongside the body, palms down. Keeping weight pressing down through the arms and through the soles of the feet, slowly roll the spine to the ground, vertebra by vertebra, until the entire back is on the ground. Relax and breathe comfortably for a few moments.

The Basic Shoulderstand
Level: 2

When you feel comfortable with the mechanics of the Shoulderstand, then try it away from the wall. The basic principles are the same except for the fact that this time you will have to lift the legs by yourself and push up as you do so, lifting the spine from the ground. Try it; if you can do the Shoulderstand against the wall, then you should certainly be able to do this one. Most importantly, remember not to move the head.

1. Begin lying flat on the back with the legs together and the arms flat down the side of the body, palms down. Relax the body and breathe normally.

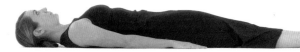

2. Contract the abdominal muscles and, with the support of the arms like levers pressing down into the ground, lift the legs off the ground and with control swing them over the head. This can be done either with straight legs or, for those who find that difficult, with the knees bent. Continue to bring the legs over the head until the lower back comes off the ground. In order to practise this movement it is beneficial to bring the legs over the head and then rest the knees on the forehead, pressing down through the arms and lifting the tailbone and buttocks high, so that the back is off the ground. Wriggle your shoulders underneath so that your shoulder blades feel as if they are coming together.

3. Bend the elbows and place the palms on the back ribcage, supporting the back. The fingers should point towards each other with the thumbs around the torso. Walk the hands down the back towards the neck in order to straighten the spine as much as possible.

4. Begin to slowly straighten the legs upward, one at a time if you wish. Push through the heels and lift the tailbone to extend the body upward.

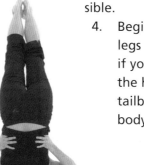

correct	incorrect
Placement of arms	

144

5. Continue to walk the hands down the back so that the elbows come closer together. The aim is to have the elbows pointing directly behind you, shoulder-width apart.

6. Gently push the chest forward so that it presses firmly against the chin.

7. In the final position the legs are vertical, together and in a straight line with the torso. The body is supported by the shoulders and back of the head. The chin is resting against the chest and the arms and hands are providing stability.

8. Relax the whole body in the posture for as long as is comfortable, focusing on the breath.

9. In order to come out of the Shoulderstand, bend the knees slowly towards the forehead then bring the legs down over the head so that they are as close to parallel to the ground as possible. (If you are particularly flexible you may take the toes all the way to the ground.) The knees may be bent if you find that the strain on the lower back or hamstrings is too much with straight legs. Release the hands from the back and place them flat along the ground, palms down and fingers spread.

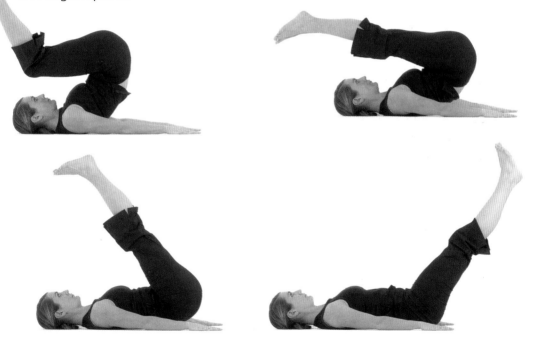

10. Slowly roll the back down onto the ground, vertebra by vertebra, pressing the hands and arms down into the ground like levers and using the legs as a counterbalance to stop you from descending too quickly. When the buttocks reach the ground, slowly begin lowering the legs down straight back to the starting position. You can also bend the legs as they go down to reduce the strain in the lower back.

11. Relax in the Corpse Pose until the breathing and heartbeat return to normal.

Beginner's variation

For those who find that they are unable to lift straight up to
the full Shoulderstand, the half Shoulderstand is a sensible option. In
this variation the back is intentionally left at a 45-degree angle to the
ground and the legs are at a right angle to the torso. The key in this variation
is to ensure that the legs remain straight to act as a counterweight to the
lower body. Visualize a jack-knife position.

Benefits: By pressing the chest against the chin this posture stimulates the thyroid
gland, balancing the circulatory, digestive, reproductive, nervous and endocrine systems, all of which combine to affect a person's weight. The thymus gland is also stimulated, boosting the immune system. Abdominal breathing is induced, improving the
flow of air. Combined with the inverted state, the blood flow is enriched. Flexibility of
the neck is increased and nerves are toned. The legs and abdomen are toned and
stagnant blood is drained from the system. Regular practice helps to prevent coughs,
cold and flu. The heart has a rest. Varicose veins are reduced. Releases tension from
the neck and shoulders. Encourages strength and flexibility of the spine.

Common mistakes: The legs are allowed to drift apart and fall down towards the
head. Keep trying to straighten directly up by lifting up through the heels and pushing
the tailbone up and forward. As much of the spine as possible should be lifted from the
ground, so keep applying pressure on the shoulders and on the back with the hands to
lift the spine from the ground. Under no circumstances should you turn the head in
either direction while in the Shoulderstand. There is enormous pressure through the
neck in the full posture and serious injury is risked by turning the head. When coming
out of the posture, do not slump the back down to the ground too quickly: take your
time and slowly bring each part of the back into contact with the ground.

Contraindications: This posture should be treated with great caution by anyone with
enlarged thyroid or high blood pressure. Those with any diagnosed back problems
should consult their doctor before attempting the posture. It should be avoided during
advanced stages of pregnancy unless under direct supervision by a qualified teacher.

Sequence: The Shoulderstand may be practised on its own or as a follow up to the
Headstand. An effective counterpose should always follow the Shoulderstand
sequence: either the Fish or the Camel. It should be practised once the body and
spine are warm

Awareness: Physical – on the control of movement, the breath or the thyroid gland.
Energetic – on vishuddhi chakra.

The Shoulderstand Cycle: Advanced Variations

There are variations to the basic Shoulderstand, which strengthen and tone the body further. Do not attempt these further variations until the basic posture is mastered. In each of the variations below it will be assumed that you have found your way into the basic Shoulderstand.

Alternate Leg Releases

This movement also acts as the next step towards the Plough and gives the hamstrings and spine a wonderful stretch.

From the Shoulderstand, exhale and release the right leg to the ground behind you, trying to touch the toes to the ground, or as close to the ground as is comfortable. Keep the left leg as straight up as possible, although beginners might find that the left leg begins to pull towards the ground as well. When the right foot has reached the ground, or as near as possible, then inhale and lift the right leg back up to the starting position. Exhale and repeat on the other side, releasing the left leg to the ground. Repeat 3–5 times, breathing slowly and moving the legs up and down in a smooth, steady way.

Abdominal Cultivation

The alternate leg releases can also be practised by releasing one leg only so far as to be parallel to the ground. This creates heat and strength in the abdominal muscles. Inhale as the leg goes down, exhale as it goes up. Repeat 3-5 times, breathing slowly and moving the legs up and down in a smooth, steady way.

Legs Wide

Doing any hip openers while inverted is a wonderful release for the muscles around the groin area. Simply go as far as is comfortable and let gravity do the rest.

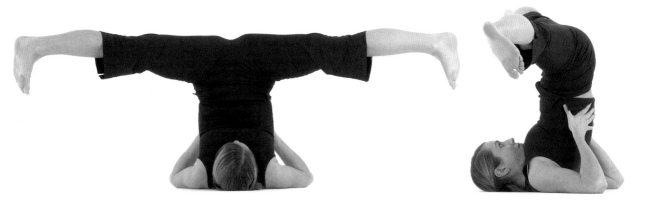

From the Shoulderstand, simply allow the legs to separate and release the feet as far as you can to either side. Maintain a straight spine throughout and try to release the legs directly out at each side, not allowing the feet to come forward closer to the head or the lower back to collapse as you open. When you have gone as far as you can go, simply remain in this position and breathe comfortably for as long as possible. You may begin to feel an extreme stretch in the inner thighs, which means you are getting the benefits of the posture. When you have stayed in the posture as long as comfortable, slowly bring the legs back together in the Shoulderstand and straighten the body back up, relaxing as much as possible.

Frog Position

In the Frog you can make a prayer position with your feet instead of your hands. This is once again a beneficial opener for the hips.

From the Shoulderstand open the legs and bend the knees, bringing the soles of the feet together above you. Press the knees back so that the hips are opened and the feet are directly above the groin area. Try to bring the heels as close to the groin as possible. Maintain a straight and erect spine throughout and breathe normally, holding as long as is comfortable. Then slowly bring the legs back together in the Shoulderstand and straighten the body back up, relaxing as much as you can.

The Candle

A candle stands tall and straight while burning and in this posture your body is also completely erect and burning internal energy. The Candle is a rigorous posture – all the weight of the body is taken by the shoulders, nape of the neck and the head. Balance is an issue in the Candle, which is why it is very important to keep your awareness focused on the upward movement of the entire body.

From the Shoulderstand, bring your legs slightly forward towards your head.

Slowly remove the hands from behind the back one at a time. While you remove the hands, test your balance and ensure that you are not going to tip out of the posture without the support of the arms. If you feel that your balance is not steady, there are two potential reasons. First, your legs may need to be further forward in order to act as a counterbalance. Second, your spinal flexibility in the basic Shoulderstand may not yet be there (so that not enough of the spine is lifting off the ground and weight is not primarily on the shoulders), and in this case it is probably best to leave trying the Candle until your Shoulderstand is much improved. However, if you find that bringing your legs further forward steadies your balance as you remove the hands, then slowly begin to lift the arms alongside the body, one at a time is sometimes helpful, fingers pointing up, until you are balancing only on the shoulders, nape of the neck and head. Pull up through the fingers and also the legs, heels and toes to straighten the body as much as possible without losing balance.

Remain in the posture as long as is comfortable, breathing normally. When you are ready, slowly place the hands behind the back again. Move back into the basic Shoulderstand.

The Shoulderstand into Bridge movement

The movement from Shoulderstand into the Bridge is a wonderful way of incorporating more than one posture into your inverted sequence. The Bridge has already been explained in the Backbending section of this book – you should be familiar with the mechanics of the Bridge before attempting this movement.

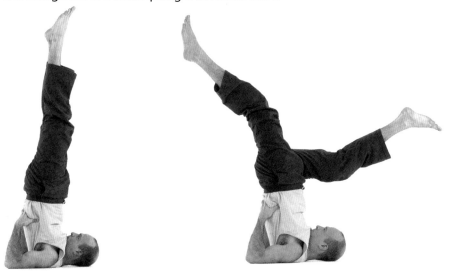

1. Begin in the basic Shoulderstand, relaxing the body and breathing comfortably.
2. Bring the right leg down towards the head so that the right thigh is parallel to the ground. The right knee may be slightly bent. Bend the left knee slightly.
3. Begin to take your left foot down to the ground in front of you, lifting your right leg naturally as a counterweight as your left foot approaches the ground. Keep pressing through the hands into the back in order to keep the arch of the lower back intact. Many students lose the arch of their lower back when they first try this movement and this makes the Bridge virtually impossible to complete.

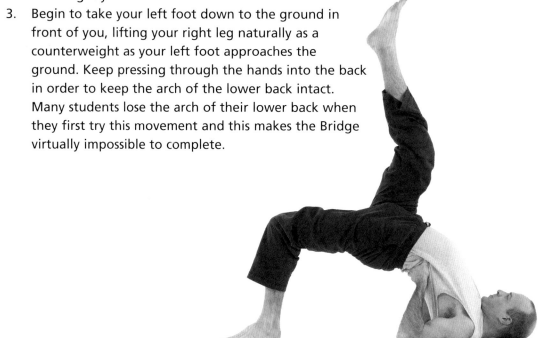

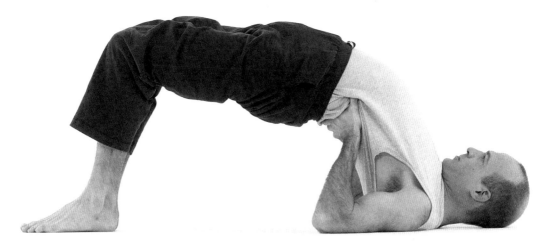

4. Keeping the back arched and the elbows pressing down into the ground, lower the right foot to the ground next to the left foot.

5. Walk the feet slightly towards you, push down into the ground through the soles of the feet and lift the abdomen and pelvis up. Adjust your hands slightly so that they are comfortably supporting your back. This is the Bridge position.

6. Remain in this position for as long as comfortable, breathing normally. If you wanted to you could come out of Bridge as normal.

7. In order to return to the Shoulderstand, press down through the right foot and upper arms and swing the left foot up into the air, lifting the abdomen back to vertical as you kick up. The natural pull of the left foot should also bring the right foot off the ground and you should continue this natural movement until both feet are vertical again, next to each other. Make any adjustments you need in order to find a comfortable Shoulderstand posture again. This movement is about courage more than anything so make sure you do a dynamic swing of the leg to assist you back up.

8. Repeat using the other foot to descend first.

The Plough Cycle

The Plough is one of the most relaxing of all yoga postures when done correctly. Many students enjoy staying in the Plough for long periods, relaxing the body and feeling the hamstrings stretch, the abdomen tone and the spine lengthen. For beginners I recommend putting a couple of pillows (or as many as you need) or even a chair behind you to put your feet on. This will assist you at first and give you a guide as to how flexible you are in the position, while also giving you the benefits of the final posture. If you find the posture simple enough using pillows or a chair, then you can move directly into the full Plough knowing it will not apply too much pressure to your back.

Although you can move into the Plough directly from a lying position by lifting the legs over the head to the ground behind you, I will be teaching Plough as part of the Shoulderstand cycle, and to go into the Plough straight from Shoulderstand. As with the variations to the Shoulderstand, I will assume that you feel comfortable in the Shoulderstand when discussing the Plough.

The Plough (Halasana)
Level: 2

1. Begin in the basic Shoulderstand, relaxing the body and breathing comfortably.
2. Pressing down on the upper arms and lifting the buttocks, slowly lower the legs over the head, keeping them as straight as possible to begin with. Try to touch the toes to the floor, but do not force them down (this is where pillows or a chair are of great help).
3. If you need to you can bend the knees slightly in order to lower the legs into a comfortable position, but remember that the ultimate aim of the Plough is to have the legs straight and toes on the ground.
4. When your toes are comfortably touching the ground, or resting on pillows or chair, then release the hands from the back and straighten the arms behind you, flat along the ground, palms down. If this is simple for you (and it will vary depending on shoulder flexibility), then you can interlock the fingers and try to press the arms and hands flat down on the ground.

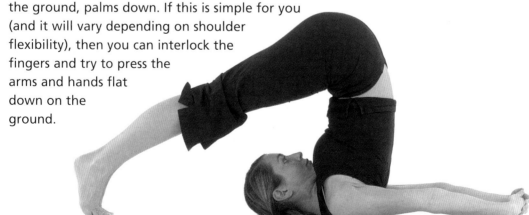

5. Continue to lift the buttocks and straighten the spine. Try to walk the toes away from you, straightening the legs by pushing up through the thighs. Relax the body and breathe easily for as long as is comfortable. It is most important not to move your head at all while practising this posture.

6. To return to the Shoulderstand, put the hands on the back to provide support for the spine and slowly lift both legs back up, preferably straight but with bent knees if necessary.

7. To come out of the Plough, place the arms down to the ground so they act as brakes as you slowly roll out of the posture, breathing naturally.

Beginner's variation

If you find that taking both legs to the ground together is difficult, you may want to bring down one leg at a time, as in the Alternate Leg Releases (see page 147). Feel free to bend your knees to help you. Or you may want to bend the knees, taking them into the forehead, then take one leg at a time behind you to the floor.

Benefits: The movement of the diaphragm during the practice of the Plough massages the internal organs and activates the digestive process, relieving constipation and revitalizing the spleen and suprarenal glands. It improves liver and kidney function, strengthens the abdominal muscles and relieves spasms in the back muscles. The spinal nerves are toned and blood circulation is increased throughout the body. The thyroid gland is regulated and the thymus stimulated.

Common mistakes: Often students allow the legs to separate and do not focus on extension of the legs and spine. Do not allow yourself to slouch into the posture, but keep pushing up through the buttocks and trying to walk the feet away from you. Continually push up further onto the shoulders, extending the spine upward. Once again, keep the head still.

Contraindications: The Plough should not be practised by anyone with slipped disc, hernia, sciatica or high blood pressure. Those with any diagnosed back problems should consult a doctor before attempting the Plough. Women in mid to late stages of pregnancy should avoid the Plough.

Sequence: If possible, perform the Plough immediately after the Shoulderstand. Follow the Plough with the Fish or Camel as counterpose. This pose should be practised when the body and spine are warm from previous postures.

Awareness: Physical – on the abdomen, the relaxation of the back muscles, the breathing or the thyroid gland. Energetic – on manipura or vishuddhi chakra.

The Plough Cycle: Advanced Variations

These variations all put tremendous pressure on the breathing and back muscles. They should not be attempted until you are comfortable in the Plough and able to take your toes all the way down to the ground with the legs completely straight.

Knees to Head Plough

From the basic Plough, bend the knees and try to place them on the ground either side of the ears, preferably touching the ears. Extend the arms behind you and wrap them over the backs of the legs, pressing the shins down into the ground. It is common for people to have trouble taking the knees to the ground, and many say that their breathing is constricted in this position. Go as far as you are comfortable and hold the posture for as long as is comfortable. If you continually work on pressing the legs down and breathing deeply, in time the knees will drop to the ground and the breathing will become easier. As soon as you feel you have had enough, simply straighten the legs and return to the basic Plough.

The Plough Forward Bend

From the basic Plough, bring the arms up over the head and try to take hold of your toes. It may be that your tailbone moves slightly back and the spine curves in order to help this movement. That is fine. Focus on straightening the legs and lifting the buttocks while in this posture. When you have stayed in the posture as long as is comfortable, lift the arms back up and return them to the ground behind you. Walk the feet away from you to straighten the spine to a vertical position and return to the basic Plough.

Wide Leg Prayer Position

From the basic Plough, separate the legs by walking the feet away from each other to either side. When the legs are opened as far as possible, bring the arms off the ground behind you and bring them up between the legs in front of you. Point your arms straight up and bring the palms together into prayer position. Maintain the lift in your buttocks and keep the toes on the ground. Continue to reach up through the fingertips and breathe normally. When you have stayed in the posture as long as is comfortable, bring the arms down and return them to the ground behind you. Slowly walk the feet back in together and return to the basic Plough.

Leg Variation in Plough

Method I
From the basic Plough, bring the hands onto the back, fingers facing each other, elbows bent so that the back is properly supported. Maintain pressure on the back throughout so that the spine stays erect. Walk both feet as far to one side as possible, keeping both shoulders on the ground throughout. Keep pushing the buttocks up and try to keep the legs perfectly straight and together. When you have gone as far as you can in one direction, remain at that point for up to 10 deep breaths, or however long is comfortable. The return to the centre and repeat on the other side.

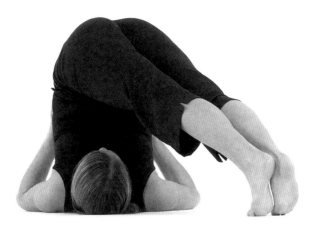

Method II
As an additional stretch in this position, try to lower both knees to the ground on one side of the head, keeping both shoulders on the ground throughout. Remain in this position for up to 10 breaths, or however long is comfortable, before straightening the legs and walking the feet back to centre.

When the feet have come back to centre, repeat to the other side.

When you have returned to the basic Plough, relax the body and breathe comfortably.

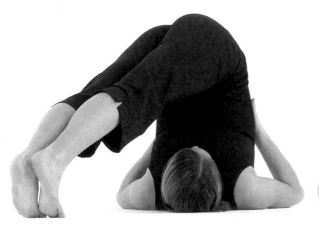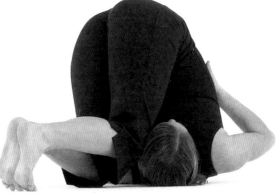

The Fish (Matsyasana)
Level: 1–2

Although not an inverted posture, more a backwards bend, the Fish is traditionally seen as the natural counterpose for the Shoulderstand cycle. I have therefore included the Fish in the inverted section, and I recommend that the Shoulderstand cycle is followed by Fish. After you have finished the Shoulderstand, you should be relaxing in the Corpse Pose, flat on your back. That is where we will begin.

1. Lie flat on your back, arms flat down by side of the body, palms down, breathing normally.
2. Bend the knee and place the foot on the ground. Roll over onto the side so that the buttock lifts from the ground, and place the arm under the side of the body, palm down and fingers pointing towards the feet. Lower the buttock onto the arm. It is extremely important to have your arms as straight as possible underneath your body to ensure that you go into the pose correctly.

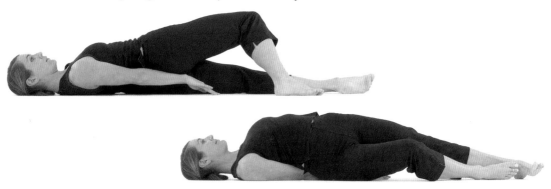

3. Now do the same to the other side so that both hands are alongside each other under the body.
4. Try to move the hands further down the backs of the legs, keeping the palms down, by bringing the elbows and shoulder blades together. This can be done by adjusting the weight to either side and pushing the fingers closer to the feet and trying to move the elbows slightly under the sides of the body. This action will help to lift the chest higher.

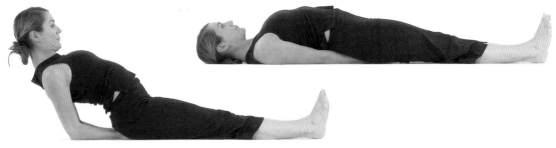

5. Pressing down through the lower arms and hands, bend the elbows and lift the upper body from the ground. The legs should remain straight and together, buttocks firmly pressing down into the ground.

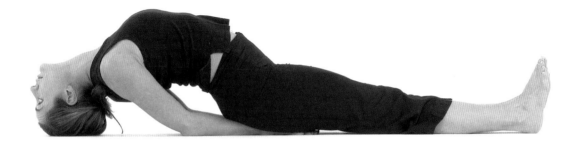

6. Arch the back and release the head down to the ground, trying to look directly behind you and finding a spot to focus on. The weight should be on the elbows, lower arms and hands, and only a little on the head. Continue to press down through the legs and buttocks and lift the abdomen and chest upwards.
7. Remain in this position for about half the length of time you were in the Shoulderstand, or as long as is comfortable. Breathe normally. Keep pressing down through the elbows, trying to move the shoulder blades together and opening the chest area further.
8. When you are ready, press down through the elbows to lift the head swiftly from the ground back into the position held in step 5. Lower the back to the ground slowly and relax in the Corpse Pose.

Benefits: This posture stretches the intestines and abdominal organs and is useful for all abdominal ailments. It encourages deep breathing and recirculates stagnant blood in the back, alleviating backache. The thyroid and thymus are both regulated and stimulated. The pelvic area is stretched and toned and shoulders and arms are strengthened. The opening of the chest and shoulders encourages correct posture.

Common mistakes: Avoid placing too much weight on the head; this can lead to possible neck complaints. Find a comfortable place to rest on the top of the head; you don't need to go too far back to get the benefits. Do not allow the legs to become completely passive, but do not tense them completely either. Keep the legs straight and together extending them away from the heels, and firm the thighs to press them down into the ground with flexed feet. Do not allow the chest to drop down, but keep lifting it throughout and use that lift to bring the elbows together underneath you.

Contraindications: Those who suffer from any diagnosed back condition should not attempt this posture before consulting their doctor. Pregnant women should only practise this posture under the guidance of a qualified teacher.

Sequence: Ideally practised after Shoulderstand and Plough as they release the neck in opposite directions, relieving muscular tension.

Awareness: Physical – on the abdomen, chest opening or breathing. Energetic – on manipura or anahata chakra.

The Fish Cycle: Advanced Variations

There are a multitude of variations for practising the Fish and I give only a few examples here. As always, you should be comfortable in the basic Fish before attempting the variations.

Prayer Position

From the basic Fish, lift the chest up as high as possible in order to alleviate weight on the elbows, and position the head so that it can support weight. When weight is removed from the lower arms, lift the arms in front of you and bring the hands together in prayer position. It is vital that you continue to press down through the buttocks, extend away from the heels and lift the chest to the sky in order that all the weight of the body is not falling down through the neck, which is exposed in this posture.

Hold the posture as long as is comfortable, breathing normally. To come out of the posture take the elbows down to the ground and move the weight of the body back onto the lower arms and hands. Then, pressing down through the elbows, lift the head and torso back up and slowly lower the entire spine to the ground.

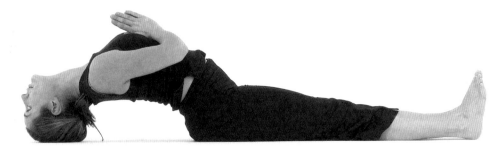

Extended Prayer Position

From the basic Fish, go into the prayer position variation as above and then lift the arms over the head to the ground behind you. It is vital that you continue to press down through the buttocks, extend away from the heels and lift the chest to the sky in order that all the weight of the body is not falling down through the neck, which is exposed in this posture.

Hold the posture for as long as is comfortable, breathing normally. Come out of the posture as before.

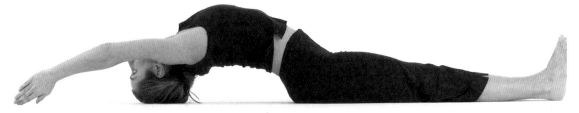

Lotus Fish

This variation should only be attempted by those able to sit comfortably in Lotus (see page 168) for long periods. Those unable to sit in Lotus could risk injury attempting this variation.

From Corpse Pose, position your arms under the buttocks as in steps 2–4 of the basic Fish. Bend the knees and cross the legs over each other into Lotus position. If you need to use your hands to move yourself into Lotus, this is of course all right: after positioning yourself in Lotus simply reposition the hands under the buttocks. Begin 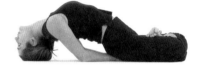 moving the legs down towards the ground. This movement lifts the lower part of the spine off the ground slightly. You may want to visualize a pendulum action, with the knees moving down as the lower back begins to lift up. Pressing down through the lower arms and hands, lift the upper body off the ground and move into the Fish position. The upper body should follow the same guidelines as for the basic Fish. Hold for as long as is comfortable. To come out of the Lotus Fish, lift the head off the ground swiftly, and, as the spine flattens to the ground, the legs will naturally lift off the ground. Begin then to unfold them from Lotus.

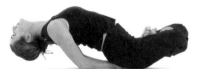 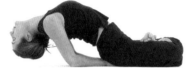

The Wall Fish

For those who want to feel their chest opening to a greater extent and to give more support to the body than the Prayer or Extended Prayer Position Fish, this variation may be beneficial.

Position yourself lying flat on your back with the wall 15cm (6 inches) behind your head. The correct distance should be where you can place the palms, fingers down, flat on the wall, with your upper arms at a right angle to the ground. Inhale and press the hands into the wall, lifting the chest and trying to keep the buttocks from sliding out. The more pressure you apply to the wall, the more you should be able to lift the heart upwards and release the head back, eventually touching the crown of the head to the ground. Stay in the position for as long as comfortable, breathing normally. To come out of the posture, lift the head and ease off the pressure against the wall, so that your back releases slowly to the ground.

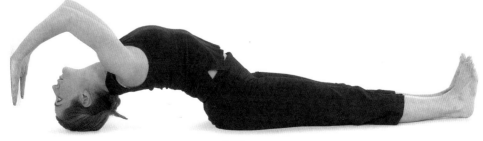

The Handstand (Adho Mukha Vrksasana)
Level: 3

The Handstand is an enormous test of strength and will-power. It requires patience to develop a solid practice and a certain willingness to try the same thing over and over again until you have the stamina to hold the position. The full Handstand is freestanding and is extremely advanced. For this reason I have decided to show versions which involve practising close to a wall, using the wall for support and balance. The benefits will be almost identical to a freestanding Handstand, with far less risk of injury and frustration. Find a wall without any artwork or hanging objects on it, as these can easily be hit by the flailing legs that sometimes accompany the Handstand. I will show you two variations to practise, both of which will develop the strength necessary to master this demanding posture. Once you have mastered the Handstand against a wall, try it freestanding: the principles are still the same, except that you must stop the movement of the legs yourself.

Beginner's Variation: Preparation for Handstand

1. Sit against a wall with the buttocks and the spine pressing against the wall. The legs are extended out in front of you, together. Relax the body.

2. Have a look where your feet are. This is the place that your hands will eventually need to go when you start this posture. Remember that spot.

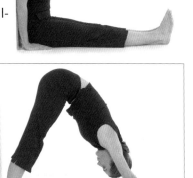

3. Now move onto your hands and knees. The hands are shoulder-width apart, fingers spread, in line with the position where the feet reached in step 2. Tuck the toes under and push the hips up into a variation of Downward Dog, with the heels against the bottom of the wall. If you find this difficult, then bend the knees. The important thing is that your hands are in the correct place, a leg's length away from the wall, and the feet are at the base of the wall.

4. Pressing down through the hands to provide a secure base with fingers spread, lift the right leg from the ground and begin walking up the wall. So long as you maintain pressure through the hands and press into the wall through the feet, you should be able to slowly walk your feet higher up the wall with complete control.

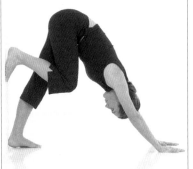 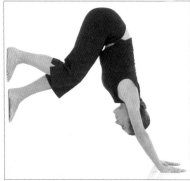

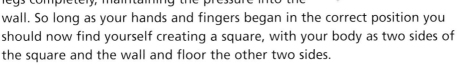

5. When you have reached the point where your legs are parallel to the ground, stop and straighten the legs completely, maintaining the pressure into the wall. So long as your hands and fingers began in the correct position you should now find yourself creating a square, with your body as two sides of the square and the wall and floor the other two sides.
6. Hold this position as long as is comfortable. Maintain straight legs and a straight spine. Allow the head to hang freely.
7. When you are ready to come out of the posture, simply walk the feet back down the wall and relax into Child's Pose for a few moments until the breathing returns to normal.

Advanced Variation: Full Handstand

1. Stand in Mountain Pose (tadasana), facing the wall.
2. Bend forward and place the palms on the ground about 30cm (1 foot) away from the wall. The hands should be shoulder-width apart and the fingers spread. Keep the arms fully stretched.

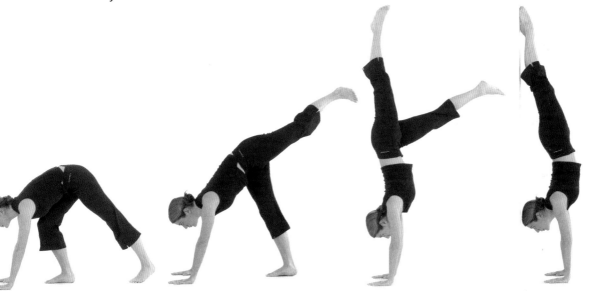

3. Take the legs back and bend the knees. Move onto the balls of your feet and press down through the hands. Exhale, and rock the body forward, swinging one leg up powerfully. At the point where the upward movement of the leg begins to lift the other foot off the ground, push off the ground with the other foot and swing that leg up as well. The legs will touch the wall one after the other

Sometimes people fail to achieve the Handstand because their hands are too far away or too close to the wall. If the hands are kept far from the wall, then the legs have further to travel in order to make contact and the resulting curvature of the spine will cause great strain. Likewise, if the hands are too close you will have to straighten the body too quickly and good balance will not be achieved.

4. Stay in the posture as long as is comfortable, breathing normally. Continue to press down through the hands and lengthen the body up through the feet.

5. To come out of the posture, push your left leg away from the wall and allow it to fall naturally to the ground. This will pull the other leg away from the wall as well and you should be able to drop to the ground gracefully, one leg after the other.

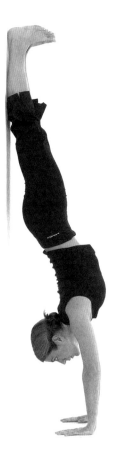

Benefits: This pose develops the body harmoniously. It strengthens the arms, shoulders and wrists and expands the chest fully. The inversion of the body reverses the blood flow and brings the benefits already discussed in the Headstand.

Common mistakes: I have already mentioned the importance of correct hand positioning. Another common mistake is bending the elbows. The arms should be kept straight throughout. The spine should not be allowed to arch but should be kept straight and strong.

Contraindications: As for Headstand.

Sequence: During any sequence of inverted postures. After you have prepared and strengthened the upper body with postures like Plank and Crow.

Awareness: Physical – on balance, breathing and the strength of the arms. Energetic – on ajna chakra.

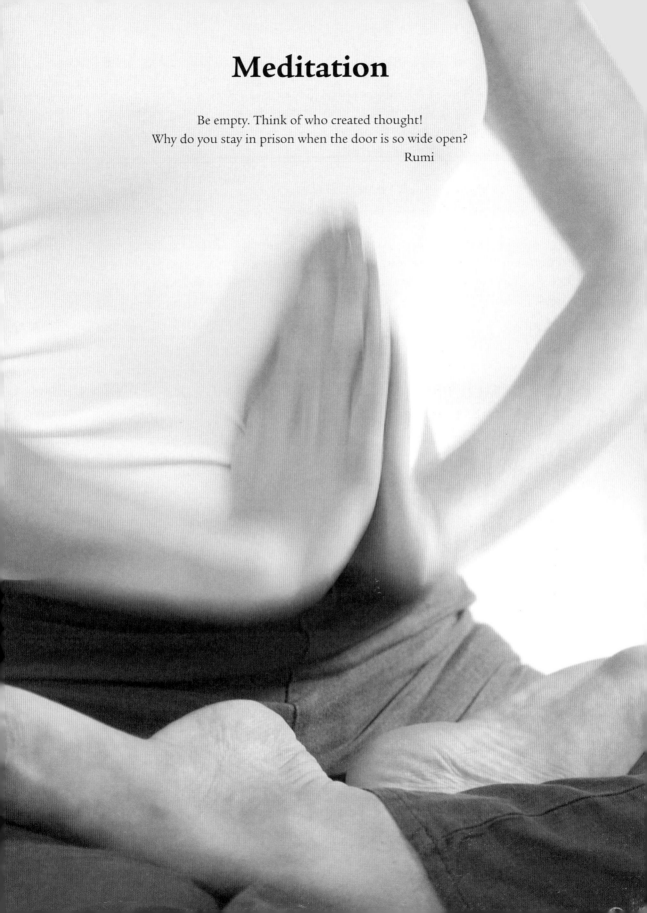

Meditation

Be empty. Think of who created thought!
Why do you stay in prison when the door is so wide open?
Rumi

...ditation is vital to the practice of yoga. However, the art of observing the mind is not something that comes naturally to many of us now. The very word 'meditation' can put some people off before they start. Let's discard any preconceptions and instead look for a moment at how our minds work, each and every moment of the day.

What was the last thought you can remember crossing your mind? Chances are it wasn't too important. Thousands of thoughts fly by every day and how many of them do you remember in a week's time? How about in a year? If we take time to listen, we may notice the almost incessant chatter of the mind.

Meditation comes with practice. It takes a bit of discipline and the desire to create some peace in the mind to allow you to see life more clearly. At first your commitment to practice may only be five or ten minutes a day. But in time you will find that the peace and happiness gained from slowing the mind down for a few minutes grows, and soon you will see the benefits creeping into everything you do.

Have you ever calmed yourself down by breathing slowly and deeply? Well, you were using the principles of meditation when you did. The breath and the mind are linked together, and observation of the breath forms the first foundation of meditation. By regulating and observing the breath, your thoughts begin to slow down and you find yourself simply observing their flow, without holding on or becoming attached to any of them.

As you continue on your journey of observation you will become aware of many different things. Your body might be stiff, or nervous, or even wonderfully relaxed. Our physical state changes from moment to moment. Through the regular practice of meditation, you will become aware of how the changes in your physical body are linked to changes in your mental state. Before too long, that increased awareness will manifest itself in everything you do. Awareness is the second foundation of meditation.

Many of you will be unused to sitting completely still, doing nothing but breathing. It may feel strange or physically uncomfortable to begin with. At first you might find yourself distracted by sounds, thoughts, smells – even sights, if your eyes are open. Don't worry about it. This is an exercise in concentration, the third foundation of meditation, and nobody is going to be perfect to begin with. Learn to focus and stay fixed on a point; the benefits of doing so will manifest themselves.

As you explore your yoga practice further, you will begin to see that the three foundations – breathing, awareness and concentration – are also the three principles underlying your practice of the postures as well. The physical postures, in time, will become moving meditations as well.

The more you practise the more you begin to understand that there is no secret method, and no quick way to mental peace. Simply by practising the techniques over time your mind begins to clear, your thoughts slow down and you are much more in control of your emotions. When that starts happening, life becomes a joy.

In my first book, I introduced three simple techniques for those with no prior meditation experience. Beginners who have trouble finding comfort in the techniques discussed here might find those covered in my first book to be easier starting points. In fact, there are hundreds of meditation techniques, and there are books dedicated entirely to explaining how to meditate. Every person is different and each of us will be stimulated by different things. If the techniques here do not do anything for you, please don't think that meditation is not for you. Meditation is for everyone, and it is just a matter of trial and error until you find the method that suits you best. All techniques have the same ultimate goal: the observation and calming of the mind. Which technique you use is up to you.

Meditation takes time and patience. The ease with which you practise meditation depends so much on what is happening in your life at that moment, physically and mentally. It is when the mind is at its busiest that meditation is most important, even if the results are not as clear as on the days when you feel serene and calm. For me, meditation acts as my brakes, slowing down my life for a few wonderful moments. I feel the benefits of that period of calm for the rest of the day. When I haven't done my daily meditation, the volume of my mental chatter gets louder and my thoughts faster. Taking just ten minutes a day to sit quietly and witness what is going on inside brings me peace and serenity to deal with what life brings my way.

Five Top Meditation Tips

1. Find a quiet, peaceful place where you won't be disturbed. Turn off all telephones and TV. Return to the same place each time you want to meditate. Familiarity is very important for calming the mind.
2. Clearly state your intention to practise for a specific amount of time before you begin. Use an egg timer or set an alarm to create a boundary for your practice so that you are not distracted by thoughts of when you should finish.
3. Make sure that the clothes you are wearing are as comfortable as the environment you are meditating in. You don't want to be too hot or too cold.
4. Choose a sitting position that is right for you from the choices I have given here. Comfort is vital while meditating. You will be sitting still for longer periods than you may be used to, and need to make sure your body isn't straining.
5. Don't try too hard. Ease and relaxation will get you further than force and frustration. Focus on the chosen technique and everything else will follow. If you drift off from your focus, gently bring yourself back.

Sitting Postures for Meditation

These sitting postures range from the simplest to the most challenging in yoga. Try them and find the one that suits you best, one you will be able to remain comfortably in. It's no good being able to do Lotus comfortably for one minute and then spending your next nine minutes of meditation in agony. Whichever position you choose, make sure the knees are below the hips, as this will assist to straighten the body. If none of these poses are comfortable for long periods, feel free to sit straight in a chair with the feet flat on the ground and the hands relaxed on each leg

Hero's Pose

This position is for people who find cross-legged poses uncomfortable.

Kneel down and sit back on the heels, resting your hands on your thighs or in your lap. Lift up through the crown of the head, straightening the spine and the back of the neck. Close the eyes and relax the whole body. Observe how you feel in this position. If you need help to make the posture more comfortable then try these props:

1. A small cushion under the arches of the feet.
2. Sitting on a cushion or folded blanket between calves and buttocks; use as many as you like.
3. Sitting on a block placed between your legs so that your buttocks are raised.

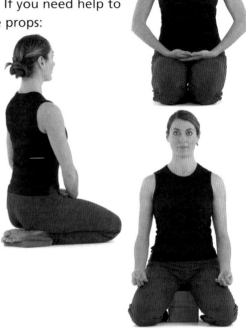

Easy Pose (Sukhasana)

Sit with the legs straight out in front of the body. Bend the legs, placing each foot under the thigh of the opposite leg. Place the hands on the knees in a comfortable position. Lift up through the crown of the head, straightening the spine and the back of the neck. Close the eyes and relax the whole body.

Easy Pose is the simplest and most comfortable cross-legged sitting position for most beginners. It brings mental and physical balance without straining the body. If you find it uncomfortable you can place a pillow or cushion under the buttocks. Place the cushion so that your tailbone is on the front edge of the pillow, tilting your pelvic area forward; you do not want to sit on the middle of the cushion. Another helpful hint is to place cushions under the knees if they are not close to the ground. Easy Pose is all about comfort and, as the name suggests, ease. Use whatever props you need to be able to relax in the posture.

Accomplished Pose (Siddhasana)

Sit with the legs straight out in front of the body. Bend one leg and place the foot under the opposite thigh, with the heel pressing on the perineum. Bend the other leg and tuck the foot into the space directly in front of the other heel, so that the heels are lined up together. The top of the foot should be on the ground and toes should face the knee. Adjust your position so that the foot feels firmly tucked in. Place the hands on the knees in a comfortable position. Lift up through the crown of the head, straightening the spine and the back of the neck. Close the eyes and relax the whole body.

The Accomplished Pose is often the most popular meditation position because it is relatively easy to feel comfortable in. By tucking the heels against each other, the lower body is held steady and this creates a base for the upper body to straighten from. If the knees are not on the ground feel free to use a cushion to support them. This pose should be mastered before moving to the Lotus position.

Half Lotus (Ardha Padmasana)

Sit with the legs straight out in front of the body. Bend one leg and place the sole of the foot on the inside of the opposite thigh. Bend the other leg and lift the foot on top of the opposite thigh. Try to place the upper heel as near as possible to the abdomen. Adjust the position so that it is comfortable. Place the hands on the knees in a comfortable position. Lift up through the crown of the head, straightening the spine and the back of the neck. Close the eyes and relax the whole body.

The Half Lotus is a preparation for the Full Lotus position. Students should not attempt to try Full Lotus until they are able to remain sitting comfortably in Half Lotus for long periods of time. If there is any strain on the body during Half Lotus then the position should not be used for meditation or any breathing exercises. The benefits of this sitting posture are similar to those of Full Lotus, though to a lesser degree.

Full Lotus (Padmasana)

Sit with the legs straight out in front of the body. Slowly bend one leg and lift the foot on top of the opposite thigh. The sole should face upward and the heel should be close to the pubic bone. When this leg is comfortable, bend the other leg and lift the foot on top of the opposite thigh. In the final posture, at least one knee should touch the ground. Place the hands on the knees in a comfortable position. Lift up through the crown of the head, straightening the spine and the back of the neck. Close the eyes and relax the whole body.

Those who suffer from sciatica, sacral infections and injured or weak knees should not do the Full Lotus. It should never be attempted until you are comfortable in the other sitting poses.

The Full Lotus is considered one of the classic poses of yoga, and there are paintings and pictures of yogis through the ages sitting peacefully in this pose. The feet press the thighs down, acting as a foundation for the entire body to straighten and be steady. The heels pushing into the lower abdomen stimulate the lower energy centres of the body, and they in turn push energy up throughout the entire torso.

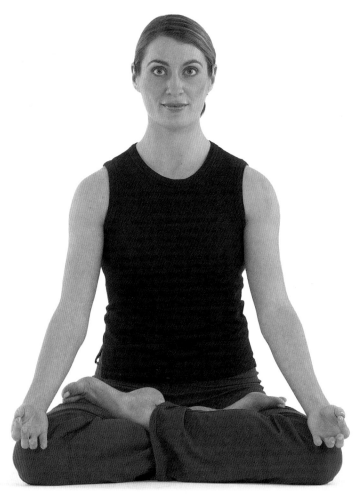

Preparation for Meditation

This preparation for meditation should be done prior to the practice of any specific technique. It acts to calm and focus the mind and body and bring the mind into the present moment. This preparation uses the full yogic breathing technique discussed on pages 22-3. Make sure you are comfortable with the art of breathing before beginning your meditation.

Sit in a comfortable position and try to straighten the back as much as possible, keeping the chin parallel to the ground so that you are looking directly forward. Place your hands comfortably on your knees or lower thighs. Close your eyes. For the next minute or so simply observe the breath. Don't try to change it or influence it, simply watch the inhalation and exhalation just as they happen. If the mind wanders then bring it back to the breath. Don't get frustrated; just relax and breathe for a few minutes using the full yogic breath technique.

Technique 1– Concentration

To begin with, the most challenging part of meditation can often be keeping the mind concentrating on the same technique for 5 minutes. How often are our minds and bodies completely still? Even in sleep the mind may be busy. Concentration is vital to meditation, as it is for many things we do. This technique is ideal for improving our powers of concentration.

Find an object on which you can concentrate. A lit candle is perfect. Place the object in front of you and sit comfortably, observing the natural breath. Look directly at the object and concentrate completely on it, trying not to blink, without forcing your eyes to stay open. Focus on every part of the object, the different colours, shapes and outlines. After about a minute of this, close your eyes and try to imagine the object you were looking at forming in the blackness between your closed eyes. Relax and see how much of the object recreates itself on your personal movie screen. After about a minute open your eyes again and concentrate on the object for another minute. Concentrate on every part of the object, then after a minute close your eyes again and once more try to recreate the image between your closed eyes. Repeat up to three times.

Gradually you will find that you are able to concentrate longer without blinking, and that the picture formed between your closed eyes becomes clearer and clearer and stays imprinted on your mind for longer. You will also find your concentration improves in everyday life.

Technique 2 – 'Painting' Meditation

Visualization is vital to all of yoga. This technique uses the art of visualization to create images within you. Think of yourself as an artist, with the body as a blank canvas and the breath as the paintbrush.

Relax the body and observe the breath. Focus on the pubic bone or bottom of the spine. As you inhale, use your paintbrush and draw a line with your breath all the way up the centre of your body to the top of the head or even higher, whether at the front, middle or back of the body. Make your breath long and flowing. Then as you exhale, follow the line back down the body with your paintbrush, making the sweep of your brush long and smooth, with the breath. Work with the movement of the breath and paintbrush up and down the body, trying to lengthen and steady the breaths. Make sure to paint every point up and down the body on that line. Continue as long as comfortable.

Now, we are going to change the shape of the painting, creating a circle with our breathing. As you inhale, begin at any point on your canvas (I usually start at a point directly in front of me) and start to paint a circle, moving slowly in whatever direction feels right to you, so that by the time you have completed a semi-circle, you are ready to start your exhalation. As you exhale, continue the circle around to the point at which you began. Continue to breathe and paint your circles, making each one slightly bigger than the last, so that an enormous swirling effect is created on your canvas. Change the colours if you wish, and vary the pace of your painting, although never the pace of your breath. For instance, if you wish to complete a full circle on your inhalation, then do so by speeding the paintbrush up – the breathing should remain at the same steady, smooth pace throughout. Continue as long as comfortable, feeling free to paint whatever you wish on your canvas. The important thing is to remain focused on the visualization and breath.

Technique 3 – Golden Thread Breath

A friend of mine practised this visualization technique while pregnant, and told me that she used it throughout her labour to amazing effect.

Relax the body and observe the breath. Try to visualize a golden thread in the space between the closed eyes. See its shape, its texture and its length. See the thread clearly. On an inhalation, visualize the thread being drawn into the nostrils. Imagine that the thread begins to spread its golden colour throughout your body, mind and soul, filling you with bright light and warming your entire being. As you continue to inhale the thread inside, more and more of the golden light flows through you. On the exhalation, imagine that you are now releasing the golden thread out of your nostrils, swirling like a corkscrew in an undulating fashion away from you into the distance until it appears to reach the horizon of the mind's eye. When your next inhalation begins, the golden thread begins to be pulled once more back into the nostrils and fresh light and warmth is brought into the body, mind and soul. Continue to inhale and exhale in this way, filling the body with warmth and clearly visualizing the movement of the thread in and out of the nostrils.

Chakras and the Energetic Body

As human beings we have both a physical body and an energetic body. If you asked a doctor of medicine what the human body was made of, he would probably say it was made up of bones, skin, muscles, etc. If you asked a yogi the same question, he would not deny that the doctor was right but would also add that the bones, skin, etc, were only manifestations of energy condensed into a human form. The energetic body is one that we cannot see or touch but it is there in each human being's make-up. It is that view of the body that I find interesting and want to explain further, more specifically the energy centres in our body known as *chakras*.

Just as the physical body is made up of a vast network of arteries and muscles connecting each part of the body to the others, so too are the more subtle layers of the energetic body connected. *Prana*, the vital energy that we all breathe in each and every moment (but which differs from the air we breathe in the same way that the spiritual body differs from the physical body), travels through our system via a network of *nadis*, or channels, (called meridians in eastern medicine) which weave their way through the body and connect all the major centres of energy: the chakras. Most ancient yoga texts speak of there being 72,000 nadis, although some claim that there are up to 350,000. It is through the practice of postures and breathing techniques that we are able to cleanse the energetic body of any blockages so the *prana* can flow freely, leaving us feeling balanced on all levels – emotional, physical and mental.

There are three main nadis, or channels, in the human body and they are all located around the spinal column.

Ida – the ida nadi begins to the left-hand side of the spinal column and coils around the central channel until it culminates at the left nostril. It is associated with the cooling energy of the body, and the moon. It is sometimes referred to as the 'comforting channel'.

Pingala – the pingala nadi begins to the right-hand side of the spinal column and coils around the central channel until it culminates at the right nostril. The pingala is associated with the heating functions of the body, and the sun.

Sushumna – the sushumna nadi is the central channel through which the life force flows and is situated along the energetic spinal column from the root of the spine to the crown of the head.

The Chakras

The chakras are energetic centres located along the channel of sushumna nadi. There are seven main chakras and each one has a specific role to play in the functioning of the body. The ida and pingala nadis coil around the sushumna nadi, passing through each one of the chakras in turn on their way to the crown of the head.

Each chakra has associated characteristics (I have named just a few). The seven chakras and their functions in ascending order are as follows.

Mooladhara chakra ('root wheel') is located at the base of the spine and is called the root chakra. When the body, mind and spirit are in balance you will feel grounded and confident.

Colour: Red

Mantra: Lam

Swadhisthana chakra ('one's own abode') can be found at the genitals. When the body, mind and spirit are in balance you will feel creative, imaginative and adaptable, and have a healthy sexual drive.

Colour: Orange

Mantra: Vam

Manipura chakra ('wheel of the jewel city') is found around the navel and corresponds to the solar plexus in the physical body. It is associated with our nervous system and its functioning. When the body, mind and spirit are in balance you will feel healthy, have initiative and courage to persevere, and are able to tap easily into your 'gut reaction' instinct.

Colour: Yellow

Mantra: Ram

Anahata chakra ('wheel of the unstruck sound') is sometimes referred to as the heart chakra, not only because of its location but also because it controls our emotional responses. When the heart chakra is open you will feel unconditional love, kindness, compassion and generosity.

Colour: Green

Mantra: Yam

Vishuddhi chakra ('pure wheel') is located at the throat. It has a hidden function pertaining to balance, not only physical but also mental balance, and the balance between giving and receiving, speech and silence, as well as a balanced metabolism. When the body, mind and spirit are in balance you will feel able to communicate freely.

Colour: Blue

Mantra: Ham

Ajna chakra ('command wheel'), which is situated in the middle of the head, is often called the 'third eye'. This chakra is the transmitter and receiver of clairvoyance, remote-viewing and other psychic activities. When the body, mind and spirit are in balance you will feel intuitive and able to access a 'sixth sense'.

Colour: Indigo

Mantra: Om

Sahasrara chakra ('thousand-spoked wheel') is located at the crown of the head and represents the uppermost chakra in both a physical sense and also a subtle energy
sense. The chakra corresponds to the ultimate level of reality and brings about the
full awakening of the enlightened state.
Colour: White
Mantra: None

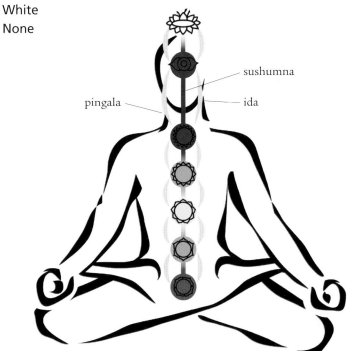

Visualization

Visualize the chakras as coloured spinning wheels of energy within you. Taking your
awareness to the chakras during meditation, breathing or practice of postures can be a
wonderful way to focus the mind on the body and the energy within. Visualizations can
be extremely powerful, but intensity varies from person to person. This is one of the last
layers to add to your practice.

Meditation on the chakras

Relax the body and observe the breath. Take your awareness to the base of the body
where the root chakra is located. Try first of all to visualize the colour associated with
the chakra, ruby red. Try to intensify this colour in your mind, then visualize it as a spinning wheel of energy at the base of your body. Stay with this visualization for a few
rounds of breath or however long your mind allows. Then continue up the body to the
next centre and colour in the same way, until you get to the crown of the head and the
final chakra. When you have finished visualizing the last colour and location, inhale then
exhale and take the breath and your thoughts back down the chakras until you reach
the base of the body to ground you.

Mudras

Happiness is a butterfly which, when pursued, is always beyond our grasp,
but which, if you sit down quietly, may alight upon you.

Nathaniel Hawthorne

The Sanskrit word *mudra* is translated as 'gesture' or 'attitude'. Mudras are psychic, emotional, devotional and aesthetic gestures. They are often associated with hand and finger positions and that is the way I will be dealing with them in this section. However, there are also mudras involving the entire body, or even just the eyes.

Mudras are said to alter mood, attitude and perception, and deepen awareness and concentration. They are said to engage certain areas of the brain and connect deeply with that area. A mudra can be used at any time, during or outside of formal meditation practice. Some people practise mudras on their own and bring specific mudras into use whenever they feel a certain need arise, and others associate them most closely with meditation and breathing techniques.

Look at mudras as a way to create a mind–body link. Since each mudra is said to have a specific function – for instance, there is a mudra to promote vitality and well-being – as you begin to form your hands and fingers into that shape you are instantly making an affirmation of intent based on that particular function. The more you do it, the stronger the link becomes, until the mind automatically begins to create positive thoughts and energy whenever you do the mudra.

Here are a few examples to try. Find a comfortable sitting position, close the eyes and hold the mudra for a few minutes. Use the affirmation suggested, or if you have a personal affirmation that feels more appropriate then go with that.

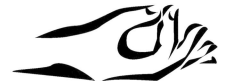 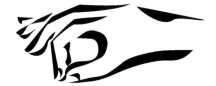

Chin Mudra and Jnana Mudra

These are the mudras of consciousness and knowledge.

Bring the index finger and thumb of each hand together. The other three fingers of each hand should be gently extended, slightly apart. Rest the hands in this position on your knees or lower thighs. If the palms are facing up, then you are in chin mudra, a passive receiving position. If the palms are facing down, you are in jnana mudra, an active giving or grounding position. (When I am in a mood to receive knowledge, to be filled up, I instinctively find my hands are more comfortable in chin mudra.) These mudras are considered to alleviate mental tension as well as promoting focus and memory.
Affirmation: My natural state is in harmony with the universe.

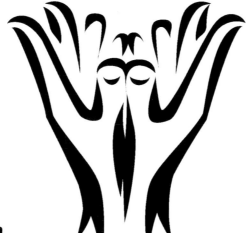

Padma Mudra

Padma is Sanskrit for 'lotus'. This mudra is the symbol of purity.

Place your hands together in front of your chest with only the edges of the hands and fingertips touching. Your hands are now in a position known as the bud of the lotus flower. If you open the hands, maintaining contact between the tips of the thumbs and the tips of the little fingers, then the flower will bloom and you will be in padma mudra. Spread the fingers wide. This mudra belongs to the heart chakra and is the traditional symbol for purity. The opening of the hands reflects the opening of the heart and mind towards our true nature and the purity of everything.

Affirmation: All is one.

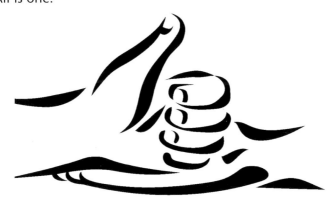

Shiva Linga Mudra

This is the energy-charging mudra.

Make a fist with the right hand and extend the thumb upwards. Place it on top of the left hand, which should be in the shape of a bowl. Position the hands at the level of the abdomen with the elbows pointing out. This mudra is done whenever we feel that additional energy is needed, whether that is because of tiredness or illness, mental or physical.

Affirmation: I am happy, healthy and whole.

The Yoga of Sound

This sound is the source of all manifestation ... The knower of the mystery of
sound knows the mystery of the whole universe.

Sufi Hazrat Inayat Khan

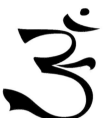

The world is vibration. All around us, at every moment, is vibration. To the yogi, the entire
universe was created by a sound – OM, the essence of all sounds, vibration in audible form.
In science as well, sound is crucial. Radio telescopy has revealed the entire universe to be
a noisy hissing vibrating symphony of sound. Since our entire universe is made up of par-
ticles of energy vibrating constantly, then sound is the most basic form of existence and
the source of all life.

In recent years scientists have shown that sound has a great effect on the growth of all
living entities. Is it any surprise that people talk lovingly to their plants to make them
grow? Or that music affects lives and can alter the mood you are in? Each of us may inter-
pret sounds differently, but the pure source of sound is the same for every living being on
the planet. In yoga, sound is a way to get in touch with the divine structure of our existence. Through sound and its vibrations we touch our innermost core.

Nada Yoga

Have you ever hummed a tune to make yourself feel better? We all use sound every day
to influence our mental well-being, and if our mental well-being is improved, so too is our
physical well-being. Yoga uses chanting in order to create vibratory changes in your state
of consciousness. Think of yourself as a radio: the chanting is to adjust the frequency to
find the clearest station. That clear station is a higher state of consciousness.

In Sanskrit *nada* means 'sound', so Nada Yoga is simply the 'Yoga of Sound'. It is the
experience of how sound vibrations, in most cases chanted and in rhythm with the breath,
affect the mind, body and spirit. The singing of hymns at church would be considered Nada
Yoga, as would humming a favourite song. As with all other forms of yoga, it is the principles of observation and awareness that make the vital difference between the act of simply creating sound and the practice of Nada Yoga.

The yogic practice of chanting is based primarily on the use of mantras. It is because
mantras are forms of sound vibration that they are so effective. There is no need to believe
in the actual truth of the mantra to receive benefits from this practice – it is the performing of the mantra and the awareness of how the sound is affecting you that is vital.

Mantra

The Sanskrit word *mantra* can be translated as 'the force that liberates the mind'. A mantra is a sacred sound. It may be an entire phrase, a single word, or even a syllable. In practice, a mantra is usually repeated one of three ways: out loud, whispered or repeated mentally. Vocalized, or out loud, is generally the easiest way to practise and experience it, and mental repetition the most subtle and meditative.

Mantras are considered to be ancient sounds that express feelings rather than concepts, emotions rather than ideas. It is said that mantras originated in the birth of language itself, and when you chant a mantra you are chanting sounds that come from the source of all life itself. Most eastern philosophies use mantra as a tool to assist in meditation. The Tibetan Buddhists chant the mantra 'Om Mani Padme Hum' constantly, and the effect on the listener can be staggering as voices and tones blend into one unique harmony, infused with emotion and flowing in tune with the breath. Experiencing such a sound in the peaceful surroundings of a Buddhist temple is enough to create a spiritual experience in even the most sceptical listener.

However, it is when *you* practise Nada Yoga, whether alone or in company with others, that the true benefits of sound can be appreciated, as you feel the vibrations throughout your entire body and hear the unique sound that only you are able to produce, made even more powerful when set against the similarly unique sounds of others. Chanting can be a joyous and uplifting experience, as anyone who has ever sung to him or herself in the shower can probably attest. And people who have been in the middle of 50,000 football fans chanting will also know the energy that can be created by our own voices. When that creation of sound is married to a complete awareness of mind, body and breath then the practice of Nada Yoga becomes every bit as beneficial as your posture practice to your entire life.

Hundreds of mantras are used for the practice of Nada Yoga. Here are just a couple for you to experiment with. One is 'OM', widely considered to be the most powerful of all mantras and one that's simple for even a beginner to chanting to appreciate. The other is a series of words associated with the chakras called the bija mantras. In both cases the best way to enjoy the experience is to sit in a comfortable position, as with meditation, and relax the body and mind. Close the eyes then go for it. Don't let your confidence get in the way of experimenting with sound; it is just your own voice, after all. This is not a singing class and there is no need to have a wonderful voice. Chanting is about the creation of sound and observing how it makes you feel. If nothing at all happens, fine, but if you let go you might just find yourself enjoying the experience. There is nothing too complicated to do. I simply hope that by following the basic instructions given here you will begin to appreciate the powerful nature of chanting and to understand what the ancient yogis meant when they said *Nada Brahma*, 'The World is Sound'.

Chanting OM

OM is made up of the combination of three syllables: 'A', 'U' and 'M'. The vibration made by each of the syllables comes from a different part of the body and you should try each syllable by itself before joining them together. First sit upright and close your eyes.

A. Inhale deeply and then simply make the sound 'A', as in 'aaahhhhh', as you exhale. The vibration will be somewhere in the region of the abdomen. Focus on that vibration for the duration of the exhalation. Inhale and repeat two more times.

U. Inhale deeply and then make the sound 'U', as in 'ooouuu', as you exhale. This time the sound should vibrate in the upper chest. Focus on that vibration for the duration of the exhalation. Inhale and repeat two more times.

M. Finally, inhale deeply and make the sound 'M', as in 'mmmmmm', as you exhale. You can make this sound with your lips sealed. The vibration should resonate most powerfully in the throat, although you may feel it in the head also. Focus on that vibration for the duration of the exhalation. Inhale and repeat two more times.

Now take a couple of slow breaths. Inhale, then open the mouth and allow the 'A' and 'U' to combine and come out as one sound, 'O', at a natural volume and tone. As you approach the end of the exhalation, close the mouth and change the sound, without stopping, to an 'M' vibration. Allow the 'M' to vibrate until the end of your exhalation and try making it longer than the 'O'. Focus on the sound, on the vibration, and on lengthening the exhalation. Take a deep inhalation and try again.

There is no limit to how many times you can repeat the chanting of OM. And there are no rules about how long to make the sound, how loud or anything else. This is your sound – feel free to experiment. Every now and again pause for a moment, breathing normally. Observe how the body and mind are feeling, and be aware of any changes.

The Bija Mantras

For each of the bija mantras, you should take your awareness and concentration to the relevant chakra during the chanting. You don't have to think of anything specific, so long as your awareness is on that area. Each mantra is to be chanted three times before moving on to the next. The sequence is always from the lowermost chakra upwards. As with the chanting of OM, the creation of sound is always done on an exhalation.

Mantra	Area of focus	Colour of Chakra
LAM	Pelvic floor	Red
VAM	Between pubic bone and navel	Orange
RAM	Solar plexus	Yellow
YAM	Heart	Green
HAM	Throat	Blue
OM	Third eye	Indigo

How to Build
Your Own Practice

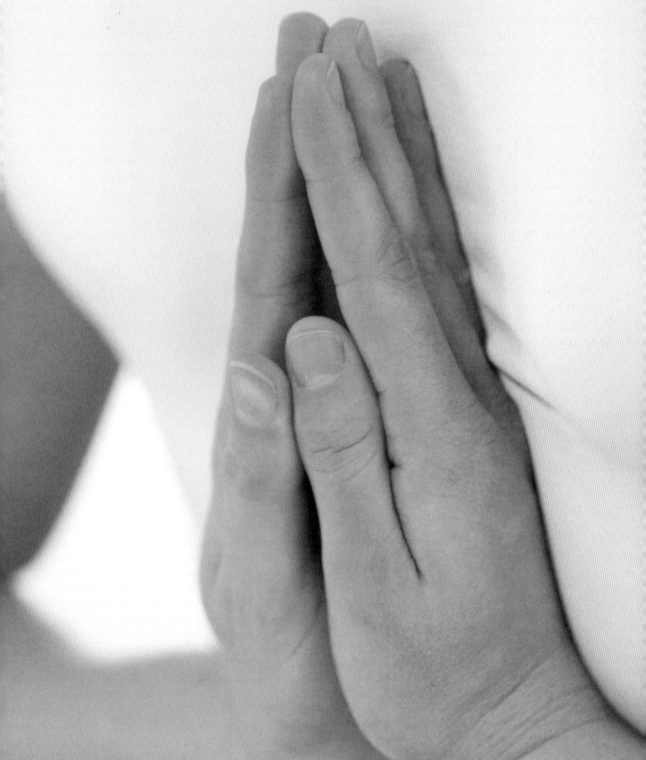

General Guidelines

Often the most challenging part for students trying to create their own practice is knowing where to start. How much time should be given to relaxation? How many postures should I do? Should I meditate before or after doing postures, or should I give meditation its own time slot altogether? These questions are normal, and have no set answers, since each of us has our own objectives and different amounts of time we can devote to our practice. But there are certainly some general guidelines you can follow to help you get started.

Q: *How much time should I give to my practice?*
A: How much time do you have? That is the first thing to be clear about. Building your own practice does not have to take away from other things you do. Everyone can make time in their day for some practice, no matter how busy. We all have routines. We wake up, brush our teeth and have breakfast. We come home from work, sit on the sofa and turn on the TV. Look at your own life and try to figure out where you can create a regular routine, even if it is only 10–15 minutes a day to start with. It is far better to do small amounts of practice every day (or every other day) than to do one four-hour session every other week. As your body and mind become used to a regular routine, it will become an accepted part of your day and you will begin to miss it if it is not there. Build slowly and try not to set unrealistic goals for yourself.

Q: *How do I fit breathing, postures, meditation, mudras and so on all into one session?*
A: You don't have to fit everything in, especially not at first. As you develop your practice you will probably find that certain things help you more than others on some days or are just more enjoyable. Understand what each limb of yoga is doing for you. If you are having a stressful week, perhaps that is a great time to spend more time on breathing and meditation to calm the mind and focus the thoughts. If you are training for a marathon, perhaps focus on postures that build strength in the legs. Have a look at the benefits for each technique and posture and decide which ones suit your own individual needs on that day. This point will be covered in greater detail later in this section.

Q: *When can I start doing the more advanced postures?*
A: Listen to and be aware of your own body and mind. As we've seen, the Sanskrit word for postures, *asana*, means 'a steady and comfortable pose'. When you honestly feel that you have reached that state in the basic (difficulty level 1) postures, then begin to experiment with the next level of postures or variations. Your own body *will* tell you if you are not ready. BE HONEST with yourself. Done properly, none of the postures should be dangerous in any way, so you can try any of them at any time. However, establishing a strong foundation, especially in the physical postures, is hugely beneficial in the long run.

Q: *Am I doing it all correctly?*

A: I have covered a lot of ground in this book, especially in respect of technique. Examine the text and pictures for each posture, and even before trying them *visualize* yourself doing them, working to understand how the different parts of your body will be moving. When you try the posture, don't push too far, and never force your body into a position it is not ready for. You could have a friend compare your technique with what is written or pictured, and ask them for some honest advice. Keep going back over the instructions, and your body will ultimately tell you whether you are doing it right or not. Relax, experiment and be aware. Remember, if you have full awareness of everything you are doing, then you are doing advanced yoga. Anyone who does things without awareness is a beginner, no matter how advanced the posture. Work on your awareness of your own body and mind constantly, and never, ever be afraid to make mistakes. Our mistakes are the greatest learning opportunities, so long as we are aware of them.

Q: *My body is aching this morning after doing yoga last night. Is this okay? Should I practise again today?*

A: Of course it's okay. Your body is telling you that you have done something active. Be aware of exactly where the aches and pains are. What postures did you do that might have contributed to them? What does that tell you about your own body's strengths and weaknesses? You are the best judge of what your body is telling you. There are no rules as to whether or not you should practise again straight away. If you want to, go ahead, but be aware of the body and make sure to warm up properly beforehand. Perhaps avoid directly targeting those sore areas with any strength-based postures. Instead, find the postures that will stretch those areas. This is what counterbalancing is all about. Sometimes something as simple as taking a hot bath will relieve the tension in your muscles.

Q: *What if I just can't do a posture?*

A: We all have different bodies. I love forward and backward bending, but sometimes my body doesn't feel comfortable upside down in a headstand. So I listen carefully on those days and respect what my body is saying. Many beginners find sitting with legs wide apart to be a challenge, or even just sitting with their back straight. You do not have to do every posture in this book to gain benefits. There will be some postures you love, and some you don't. Some will come naturally to you, and others will feel uncomfortable and alien. This is what body awareness is all about. Know your limitations, but challenge your limitations too. Find a posture you aren't drawn to and spend time every week exploring it.

Q: *Do I need to go to any group yoga classes as well?*

A: You don't need to. This book is about encouraging you to create your own home practice, and giving you the tools to do so. But group classes are a great way to pick up ideas about sequencing, and to see how different teachers explain postures. If you can find a qualified teacher you are comfortable with, it is also a great way to get your own technique corrected.

Building a Class

Most classes follow a set layout, no matter who the teacher is or what the style of yoga is. The actual sequence can vary from class to class, teacher to teacher, and method to method, but the general layout usually stays the same.

1.   Initial Relaxation
2.   Warm-up
3.   Sun Salutation
4.   Postures
5.   Breathing
6.   Meditation
7.   Final Relaxation

It is as simple as that. Some yoga methods, Sivananda Yoga for instance, do the breathing techniques after initial relaxation – but, in the case of Sivananda, that was only because its creators found that some students, just interested in the postures, would walk out before the end of the class and miss the breathing techniques. The Ashtanga method of teaching does very little in the way of gently warming up the body, instead preferring to go straight into their sequence of postures. Iyengar and Bikram classes generally do not do the Sun Salutation at all. There will always be small differences between styles of yoga, but the above should work well as a general guideline. You don't have to include all of the above in your practice every day.

   At the end of this section is a chart of all the postures covered in this book, which gives a page reference and lists which parts of the body the pose will benefit. So if your shoulders and neck are stiff after a day at your desk you can quickly see which postures will stretch these areas. Or if you want to work on strengthening your legs, for instance, you can find the postures that will most benefit you. I hope you find this a useful guide when it comes to building your class

Initial Relaxation

Always start your practice with a period of rest and relaxation, even if only for a few minutes. This should be used to bring your mind and body to the present moment, away from work, or dreams, or the thought of everyday life. Just relax and begin to be aware of how the body is feeling. Clearly acknowledge your intention for your practice. Dedicate this time to you, and no one else. Come home to yourself. Take a moment to connect to your life, to observe your own body and mind. Ask yourself these questions:

1.   How is my body feeling right now? Wait for an honest answer.
2.   How would I describe my mind in a word at this point in the day? Wait for an honest answer.
3.   How has my emotional state been today? Wait for an honest answer.

Warm-up

Warming up for a yoga session uses the same principles as warming up for a jog or a game of tennis. It is about loosening up the different joints in the body before moving into specific postures. My first book, *Introducing Yoga,* explains this, if you are unsure how to warm up. However, just think about stretching each part of the body in turn, making sure that you cover all the major muscles and joints. Start at the bottom of the body and move up. The less flexible you are to begin with, the more time you should spend warming up the body. There is nothing wrong with beginners using their entire practice to warm up, if they honestly feel that for the moment the postures may be too challenging. Often this is the case for people who have just recovered from surgery; a period of time is needed for the body to gain movement again.

Sun Salutation

The Sun Salutation is actually considered a warm-up sequence. For many students it is their only means of warming up the body. But this sequence is much more than just a warm-up; it can also be an entire practice by itself. The most important thing is to learn the sequence properly to begin with. In fact, I recommend to beginners that practice time after warm-up is spent just moving through the Sun Salutation and understanding how it flows and linking the breath with movement. You have got to start somewhere, and this is a good place. Just learning the sequence is a great workout, as your body will be moving in different directions, up and down, back and forward. As you gradually become more confident doing the sequence, and have memorized the entire flow, then you can bring it into your practice in different ways:

After your warm-up. Initially I recommend that beginners still warm up the body for a while before starting the Sun Salutation. It is an intense sequence and involves a few deep stretches so make sure you are ready. Warm up the body properly and then do two or three full rounds. You can always do more if it is comfortable.

Instead of your warm-up. This should be an option only for those students who are comfortable with the entire flow of the sequence and whose bodies can handle it at the beginning of their class. Once again, two or three full rounds are enough, but five or six will make your body really feel the difference, as with this number you begin to deepen and coordinate the breathing with the movement and heat the body.

As your entire practice. It is not uncommon for students to do nothing else but the Sun Salutation in their session. There is no maximum number of rounds you can do. You can move as quickly or as slowly as you want, and even hold postures for long periods of time. Once again, however, this option should be considered only once you are comfortable with the sequence. But, by all means, experiment with pace, duration and intensity. The magic number for the amount of Sun Salutations is 108. A friend of mine has done this amount in one go and it made him feel unbelievable, so if you have a spare couple of hours, go for it!

As a sequencing link for other postures. This option is for those who not only are comfortable in the Sun Salutation, but also are comfortable in a majority of the basic postures. What is the Sun Salutation but a sequence of postures brought together by the breath? There is nothing to stop you bringing in other postures where you see that a natural progression from one to the other exists. For instance, when you bring the right/left leg forward in step 9 of the sequence, you are in a natural position to turn the back foot out and straighten the body up into Warrior I, Warrior II, Triangle and so on. The Downward Dog (Inverted V) is another great one to use as a bridge to other postures, and I will be discussing this more later. As you become comfortable with the postures, you may begin to see natural links yourself. Experiment – know that so long as your awareness is there, everything you are doing is right.

Postures

Beginners should concentrate on postures with a difficulty rating of 1. Even those of you who have done yoga before should spend time ensuring you are completely comfortable in the basic postures before proceeding. Try not to fit as many postures as you can into a session. If you have only 15 minutes, then just pick three to five and really take your time discovering how they feel in your body. Understand how to move into the postures and how to move out of them. How you get in and out of a posture is as important as holding the pose itself. It is no good being perfect in a pose if you then injure yourself moving out of it too quickly. So what postures should you choose? First answer these questions:

Q: *How much time do you have?*
A: Obviously, the more time you have, the more postures you can choose. Make sure you take into account relaxation, warm-up, Sun Salutations, and whether or not you will be doing breathing techniques and meditation. If you have 15 minutes, pick three to five postures to work on, 30 minutes then six to ten, and so on. Make sure to take the difficulty ratings into account. If you are trying a more advanced posture for the first time, give yourself extra time to experiment with it.

Q: *What is your intention for your practice?*
A: If you have something specific to work on, for instance, tension in the neck and shoulders or tight hamstrings, then pick postures that stretch or strengthen those specific areas. If you want a general workout, then choose a couple of postures from each section: standing, sitting, backward bending, inversions. Or just concentrate on standing postures. However, if you are concentrating on backward bending, make sure the body is really warm from previous postures and you must include counterposes (twists, followed by some gentle forward bending) to balance your body. More on that subject next.

Q: *What order should they be in?*
A: Once you have decided on a number of postures to try, there are some general rules for sequencing.

1. Think long-term, not just today. Always create one day's practice with the next in mind. What do you want to achieve over a period of time? If you want to work on your leg strength and flexibility, then think about a programme over a month or two that will gradually work on each part of the legs. Keep extending your time frame forward. Remember that just because you want to work on one part of your body it doesn't mean that you ignore other postures. Try to bring balance to your planning while still focusing on your original intention.

2. Remember the spine. All yoga postures affect the spine in one way or another. It is the central structure of our skeletal frame and needs to be looked after. When thinking about sequencing, visualize the spine and try to bring in postures that move and stretch the spine in each direction, not just forward, but also back and to the sides. However, you may do backward bends after forward bends, but try not to do forward bends immediately after backward bends. The stretch of the spine in a forward bend is a lengthening that follows the natural curvature of the spine. A backward bend compresses the spine more than it lengthens it as it often works against the curvature of the spine. The pressure on the vertebral discs, which are between each vertebra, is much more intense in a backward bend. Therefore, to follow a backward bend with a forward bend can put extreme pressure on the discs and spine. Follow a backward bend with a twisting posture or with a relaxing forward movement, such as Child's Pose, before attempting a deeper forward bend. Inversions for beginners should be at the start of their practice. This is simply because of the effort required in Inversions. Intermediate students more confident in their capabilities and strength may feel free to place inverted postures wherever they choose, as long as they remember to leave themselves plenty of energy to experiment with these strong but beautiful movements.

3. Stretch, then strengthen. Ensure that postures are placed in such an order that specific muscles are stretched and loosened before attempting postures that will strengthen those muscles. For example, in standing you may wish to place Triangle, which stretches and tones the legs, before Warriors, which strengthen. Use the warm-up to concentrate on muscles that you will be working on to ensure they are properly stretched and warm. For example, with Triangles and Warriors, you can see and feel that it is working on the pelvic area and inside thighs – the Butterfly and Cradling Lotus would be gentle hip openers to start the work on those areas.

4. Start strong, end soft. Standing postures are regarded as some of the most demanding postures, which is why they are often placed at the start of classes. On the other hand, sitting or lying postures may be considered 'soft' postures, because they are non-weight bearing and require less effort. Based on this principle, you can see why inversions should be first for a beginner. More advanced students often do them at the end of practice as they are comfortable with these poses and they require

minimum effort. Do not end with a twisting posture. These postures give a one-sided stretch to the spine, and so it is always advisable to counter them with a forward movement, such as a sitting or standing forward bend, or simply drawing the knees into the chest and holding them to realign the spine from the twist. Listen to your body. Whenever you need to rest, either choose a relaxation posture that is suitable for the location your body is in (for instance, if you are on your front doing backward bends, then relax by lying on your front rather than coming up into standing to relax) or choose the position you are most comfortable in. Feel the relaxation. Rest. Close your eyes and breathe. Be creative.

So long as you follow the general guidelines above, feel free to create your own sequences. The Downward Dog (Inverted V) is a great linking posture. For instance, visualize the following sequence: Downward Dog – Triangle – Downward Dog – Warrior I – Warrior II – Downward Dog – Standing Forward Bend – Downward Dog – Cat – Downward Dog. Think about how stepping one leg at a time from Downward Dog, or dropping to your knees from Downward Dog, would make this sequence flow together (remembering to do both right and left sides of the body). Take your time and think about it. You may not be able to see the flow immediately, but as you become familiar with the postures, and especially the part of the Sun Salutation where you step forward with one leg from Downward Dog, you should begin to see how different postures are able to link together. View it as a yoga dance. Try to listen to how your own body wants to move. And remember, the Mountain Pose and the relaxation poses are postures in themselves, and therefore are also linking postures and require just as much awareness as the 'normal' postures.

Q: *What is a counterpose?*
A: A counterpose is a posture that will balance the body back to neutral. For example, backbends are primarily very stimulating in nature so you would want to counter them with seated lying twists, hip openers or some abdominal strengthening.

Q: *Can I start now?*
A: Of course. Have fun!

Breathing

Although some forms of yoga practise breathing techniques at the beginning of the class, it is more common, and traditional, for breathing techniques to be done at the end of a class, after the postures. As the postures loosen the body, they open the air channels and relax the muscles. This should make breathing clearer and easier. You may also choose simply to do breathing techniques and nothing else during a session. That is fine, and can be incredibly rewarding in itself.

Meditation

Meditation should be after your physical work, when the body has been loosened and the mind is relaxed and ready to move into quiet. I have often found that using a particular breathing technique to focus my mind helps to bring me to a quiet and peaceful state in preparation for meditation. Chanting also helps me to find a calmer state internally. In this way I am less likely to fidget and more willing to sit for long periods. However, once again, you may choose to make your own time to practise meditation and nothing else.

Final Relaxation

Don't rush to get up and get on with your day after you finish your postures, breathing, meditation, etc. Take time and observe what your practice has brought to you. Give yourself five to fifteen minutes, depending on the total length of your practice, to enjoy nothing more than just lying down breathing and relaxing. Often, when you allow yourself this pleasure, you won't want to get up after a while! This is one of my favourite parts of my daily practice. Make sure to go through the body and observe it during relaxation. Be aware of how it feels. Like at the beginning of your practice, ask yourself the following questions, this time to see the changes that might have been brought about from practising yoga.

1. How is my body feeling right now? Wait for an honest answer.
2. How would I describe my mind in a word at this point in the day? Wait for an honest answer.
3. How has my emotional state been today? Wait for an honest answer.

How have your answers changed during the course of your practice? Have they changed at all? Be honest.

And finally ...

You wondered where you could bring chanting and mudra into your practice? Well, here is your chance. Take a moment after final relaxation to sit in a comfortable position and choose a mudra for your hands. Relax, close your eyes and take a deep inhalation, then, as you exhale ... chant om three times

OM, OM, OM

Move your hands into prayer position in front of your heart and bow down to the teacher that is within you.

Thank yourself for your patience, perseverance, observance, awareness, and just for connecting to who you really are.

Lift the corners of your mouth. Smile.

Namaste. (Namaste translates loosely as 'my soul meets your soul'. Such a beautiful thought).

NAME	SANSKRIT NAME	PAGE	LEVEL (1,2,3)	PHYSICAL AWARENESS	ENERGETIC AWARENESS
Sun Salutation	Surya Namaskar	35-42	1-3	Flow	Various
STANDING					
Mountain Pose	Tadasana	44	1	Poise & Alignment	None
Tree Pose	Vrksasana	45-6	1	Balance	Anahata
Eagle	Garudasana	47	2	Balance	Mooladhara
Fierce Pose	Utkatasana	48-9	1	Strength in Legs	Anahata
Warrior I	Virabhadrasana I	50-1	1	Lift & Strength	Anahata
Warrior II	Virabhadrasana II	52-3	1	Strength & Stillness	Mooladhara/ Manipura
Warrior III	Virabhadrasana III	54-5	2	Balance & Extension	Manipura
Triangle	Trikonasana	56-7	1	Movement & Balance	Manipura
Reverse Triangle	Parivrtta Trikonasana	58-9	1-2	Movement & Balance	Manipura
Standing Forward Bend	Uttanasana	60-3	1	Pelvic area	Swadhistana
Wide Leg Forward Bend	Prasarita Padottanasana	64-7	1	Pelvic area	Swadhistana
Extended Side Angle Pose	Utthita Parsvakonasana	68-9	1-2	Extension & Balance	Manipura
Half Moon Pose	Ardha Chandrasana	70-71	2-3	Balance & Lift	Anahata
Standing Split-leg Stretch	Parsvottanasana	72-5	2	Balance & Extension	Swadhistana
Cresent Moon	Anjaneyasana	76-9	1	Lift & Stretch	Swadhistana/Vishuddhi
Side Leg Stretch	Skandasana	80	1	Balance & Length	Mooladhara/ Anahata
FLOOR					
Staff Pose	Dandasana	82	1	Poise & Alignment	N/A
Seated Forward Bend	Paschimottanasana	83-4	1	Extension & Fold	Swadhistana
Butterfly	Baddha Konasana	85	1	Relax & Open	Mooladhara/ Swadhistana
Single-leg Forward Bend	Janu Sirsasana	86-7	1	Extension & Fold	Swadhistana
Inclined Plane	Purvottanasana	88-9	1	Lift & Length	Manipura
Cradling Lotus	N/A	90-1	1	Relax & Lengthen	Mooladhara/ Swadhistana
Seated Wide Leg Forward Bend	Upavitha Konasana	92-3	2	Open & Lengthen	Mooladhara/ Swadhistana
Double Pigeon	Dwi Pada Rajakapotasana	94-5	3	Relax & Open	Mooladhara/ Swadhistana
Cow's Face	Gomukhasana	96-7	3	Relax & Extend	Mooladhara/ Swadhistana
Half Spinal Twist	Ardha Matsyendrasana	98-9	1-2	Twist & Stretch	Manipura
Downward Dog	Adho Mukha Svanasana	100-101	1-2	Lift & Extension	Vishuddhi
Crow	Bakasana	102-3	2	Balance & Strength	Anahata
Side Angle Crow	Parsva Bakasana	104	2	Balance & Strength	Anahata
BACKWARD BENDING					
Cobra	Bhujangasana	106-7	1	Movement & Arch	Swadhistana
Locust	Shalabhjansana	108-11	2-3	Abdomen & Back	Vishuddhi
Bow	Dhanurasana	112-13	1-2	Abdomen & Back	Vishuddhi/ Anahata/ Manipura
Camel	Ushtrasana	114-15	2	Abdomen, Throat & Spine	Swadhistana/ Vishuddhi
Cat	Marjari-asana	116-17	1	Breathing & Flexion	Swadhistana
Bridge	Setu Bandhasana	118-21	1	Abdomen & Flexion	Vishuddhi/ Anahata
Wheel	Chakrasana	122-3	3	Relaxation & Chest Opening	Manipura
Lying Spinal Twist	N/A	124-7	1	Length & Rotation	Manipura
INVERTED					
Dolphin	N/A	130	1	Abdomen & Breath	Manipura
Headstand	Sirsasana	132-5	2-3	Balance & Breathing	Sahasrara
Supported Headstand	Salamba Sirsasana	136-7	3	Balance & Breathing	Sahasrara
Scorpion	Vrischikasana	138-9	3	Balance	Ajna
Shoulderstand	Sarvangasana	141-51	2	Movement, Control & Thyroid	Vishuddhi
Plough	Halasana	152-5	2	Abdomen & Relaxation	Manipura/Vishuddhi
Fish	Matsyasana	156-9	1-2	Abdomen, Chest & Breath	Manipura/Anahata
Handstand	Adho Mukha Vrksasana	160-62	3	Balance, Breathing & Strength	Ajna

SHOULDERS		ARMS		WRISTS		LEGS		ANKLES		HIPS & BUTTOCKS		STOMACH & WAIST		CHEST		BACK		NECK		BALANCE	SPINAL TWIST	CONCENTRATION
Stretch	Strengthen	Stretch	Strengthen	Stretch	Strengthen	Stretch	Strengthen	Stretch	Strengthen	Stretch	Strengthen	Stretch	Strengthen	Stretch	Strengthen	Stretch	Strengthen	Stretch	Strengthen			
X	X	X	X	X	X	X	X	X	X	X	X	X	X	X	X	X	X	X	X			
PREPARATION & RELAXATION																						X
						X	X		X	X										X	X	X
X						X	X	X	X											X	X	X
X	X							X	X	X		X										
X	X			X				X	X	X	X	X		X		X						
X	X					X		X	X	X	X		X			X		X				
X	X					X		X	X	X			X			X				X	X	X
						X	X	X	X	X	X	X	X	X		X				X		
X	X					X	X	X	X	X		X	X	X		X		X		X	X	X
						X	X	X		X			X	X		X	X					
						X	X	X		X	X		X	X		X	X					
	X					X	X	X	X	X	X	X										
X						X	X	X	X	X			X	X						X		X
						X	X	X	X	X	X	X				X				X		
X	X					X	X	X	X	X	X	X				X	X	X	X	X		
						X	X	X	X	X	X									X		
PREPARATION & RELAXATION																						X
						X				X		X		X	X							
						X				X												
						X				X		X		X	X							
X	X		X		X			X		X		X		X		X		X				
										X												
						X				X		X	X			X						
						X		X	X	X	X					X						
						X				X	X											
						X				X		X	X	X		X	X	X			X	
X	X	X	X	X	X	X	X	X	X	X	X	X	X	X	X	X	X					
X	X		X	X	X					X				X		X				X		X
X	X		X	X	X					X				X		X				X		X
	X		X		X			X		X	X	X	X	X	X	X	X	X	X			
	X		X						X	X	X	X		X		X	X	X	X			
X	X	X				X	X			X	X	X	X	X		X	X	X	X			
X	X		X	X	X	X				X	X	X	X	X		X	X	X	X			
	X			X	X					X	X	X		X	X	X	X	X	X			
X	X					X	X			X	X	X		X		X	X	X				
X	X	X	X	X	X	X	X	X	X	X	X	X	X	X	X	X	X	X	X			
X		X								X		X	X	X		X	X	X			X	
	X		X									X		X		X		X				
	X		X									X		X		X		X	X	X		X
	X		X	X	X							X		X		X		X	X	X		X
X	X	X	X			X	X			X		X	X	X	X	X		X	X	X		X
X	X		X		X					X		X		X				X	X			
X	X	X				X		X		X				X		X	X	X				
X	X		X									X	X		X	X	X	X				
	X		X	X	X							X	X	X		X	X	X			X	X

189

Final Thoughts

Writing this book has been an extraordinary experience. The process has taken me on an exciting adventure and opened to me an undiscovered side, which I welcome with open arms.

I hope its pages bring you as much discovery and pleasure as writing it has brought to me. I hope that it brings you more than you may have intended when you purchased it. Something unexpected, special, a chance to look inside yourself and truly know that you have returned home. Too many of us spend our days looking externally for answers, when all along the peace we crave is within. Yoga can take you there . . . all you need to do is let it.

I would like to extend my deepest and most sincere thanks to a few people who have been on this adventure with me.

Firstly, Paul, Mr Collins, who listened to me, talked to me and inspired me further and further to reach these pages you read now. Without you, Paul, your work and dedication to this book, I would have been running a marathon. Instead, I floated on angel's wings.

To the beautiful Michael Hallock, whose help at the last hurdle was a must! I can't thank you enough. Om.

To Jim Marks, who captured such beautiful photos. Dazzy and Katie, for their obvious talent in the 'beauty beauty' department, and to Ingrid at Macmillan for sending me that email. To all my loving family and friends on this plane or higher, to whose souls I send eternal peace. I bow at your lotus feet.

Finally, to my teachers and students, who make my heart shine each moment of each day. I'm honoured and blessed to be at your side.

Yoga brings different things to everyone. In preparing for this book, I asked some of my students to say a few words about how yoga has affected their lives. I am not saying you will have the same experience, but . . .

'Yoga gives me both the energy and the inner peace I need to deal with being a mum to my eight-month-old boy. It's my time to become grounded, sane and peaceful.'

Josie Alonso, Australia

'I have been a student of yoga for just over a year now. In that time, I have experienced life-changing results, both physically and mentally. I could not assign a value to the sense of well-being and self-confidence that yoga has given me.'

Holly Bannon, Los Angeles, USA

'I have been practising yoga for a short time now and on a regular basis. It has made me suppler, more relaxed, my thoughts are clearer, and I see yoga becoming part of my life. After only about twenty minutes per day over about three months I discovered that I could twist further, bend further, breathe better, and guess what . . . there was no pain! I used to run half marathons and really pound the gym but I developed RSI injuries, so I see the relaxing postures of yoga as being really beneficial. I still go to the gym but approach it in a more relaxed way, less competitively and less intensely. I look forward to the places that yoga will take me to and the unknown but positive changes that it will induce.'

Paul Mortimer, England

'At times, being a homeopath can feel like I have to be all things to all people. Yoga brings me back to the essence of my true self. It provides me with insight, enlightenment and peace in my normally hectic lifestyle. Practising yoga for me is my special time, my safe place, where I can just be.'

Marilyn Casey, London, England

'Yoga is so unlike anything else I've tried that I became a convert quite quickly. Modern life is so busy and rushed, but going to a yoga class is the one time I stop each week and take time out to focus on myself. It has made me so much more aware of my breathing, posture, strength and balance that it's opened up new possibilities of where my body and mind can find space to relax and re-energize.'

Lynn Buchanan, Scotland

'As a relative newcomer to yoga it has given me a sense of inner calm and tranquillity, combined with a yummy sensation of stretching and working with my body.'

Wendy Longman, London, England

'When I started yoga, my energy levels were quite low. I was quite stressed and giving a lot of myself to others without being able any more to find ways of replenishing myself. Yoga has taught me how to give while receiving at the same time. I have often dedicated my classes to members of my family or friends in need . . . I believe in a kind of telepathy. Lately, I've been dedicating the classes to myself to find renewed strength. I look forward to my class, knowing that it will rebalance me, my body and my soul, that it will calm me down.'

Laurence Batista, France

About Katy Appleton:

I trained as a ballet dancer from an early age with the Royal Ballet School and English National Ballet School and then spent eight years dancing professionally around the world, with some of the major ballet companies. It seemed a natural progression to me from dance to yoga and in 1998 I became qualified to teach.

Having been a dancer I have found that this has given me an extra ordinary vision on how bodies move which has been invaluable to my students and me, especially with their posture and alignment. I'm a Sivananda trained teacher but I tend to fuse some of the physical methods together (Ashtanga, Iyengar, Sivananda) to suit the person I'm working with. I run yoga classes in south-west London and you can find details on my website.

Contact Appleyoga:

appleyoga, PO Box No 32934, London SW19 6FB

t: +44 (0) 20 8788 8892

www.appleyoga.com e-mail: katyana@appleyoga.com

Also available from Pan Books:

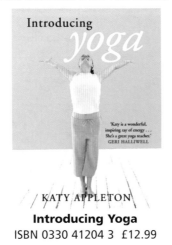

Introducing Yoga
ISBN 0330 41204 3 £12.99

I have also created two videos with Geri Halliwell available at all good video/DVD stockists.

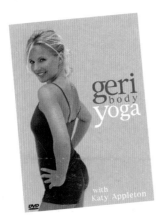

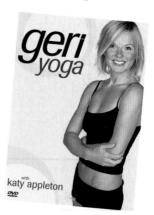